JOSEPH BOSILJEVAC, MD, PHD, FACS

Survival on an Island

Health and Immunity from the Epicenter: A Doctor's 2020 Journal

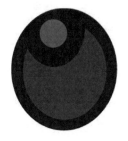

First edition

ISBN: 978-1-7357217-1-2

Editing by Corbin Bosiljevac
Cover art by Dan Ferrell

This book was professionally typeset on Reedsy.
Find out more at reedsy.com

*For John Mallon who taught me to think outside the box
and my son who taught me serenity.*

Contents

III   Part Three

IV   Part Four

Foreword

By Dr. Joseph Bosiljevac

Practicing surgery for 29 years near Kansas City was a pleasant way to begin my career. Now pushing 70, I have called The Island of Manhattan home for 12 years. The move to New York was the start of another adventure in my life that has brought on an interesting twist recently. I quickly realized that this pandemic is bigger than the Vietnam War and 9/11. This will be a major exploit and it is just starting. Subsequently there will be far reaching economic consequences. Herein lies an account of this historic event from the epicenter, my island on the east coast of the United States of America.

My conventional medical training was in general and cardiovascular surgery. I also have a doctorate in natural medicine and have experiences with alternative treatment methods.

Moving to New York in 2008 to open and age management practice was a big step for me. With this practice I found that body parts wear out and I became involved with some retired NFL and NBA players doing stem cell treatments, mostly on deteriorated joints.

I also started to see military special forces members. Besides joint and soft tissue injuries I began using systematic treatment with stem cells for lung issues, autoimmune conditions, traumatic brain injury and multiple sclerosis. My surgical background enabled me to be well acquainted with wound care principles.Used together with stem cell treatments in an overall program has markedly improved results of treatment.

There are two goals in this communication.

One is from a physician standpoint. I am living in the New York City epicenter. By means of regular emails to my patients and articles published on a regular basis I try to educate individuals on good health practices. Immune Boosting treatments are of high interest in recent months and should be for the foreseeable future.

The second is that I also live here so I can provide a citizen standpoint. Social distancing is the most beneficial method to stay ahead of this pandemic. This term is evolving to become a social norm rather than a temporary practice.

There is a medical challenge for treating the virus but also a social aspect to contain a pandemic involving our entire nation. What we learn today will help us battle future infections.

I am not a native New Yorker. Still, listening to feedback from patients over the last 12 years has enlightened me. The consequences of this pandemic are worse than 9/11. There has already been an incredibly significant economic slowdown - almost stopped.

My concerns about coronavirus began in the early part of March. From a physician standpoint I continue to follow news and review medical information. The following manuscript is a short journal and some photos of Manhattan during the current pandemic. It will give an idea of how attitudes and actions progress during the disaster. Initially experts thought it to be a bad flu, but it appears not to be highly contagious. It started in China in November and there was foreign travel prior to when the Wuhan epidemic came to light.

By the end of April, health orders were extended with general predictions on social distancing and reassessment in the plans. Finding a vaccine, altering business practices to get the economy moving, and learning what our new approach to health will look like are the stir among the American people. From my view, we follow the pandemic patient to make the next decision depending on what is evolving clinically. It is the only way health care professionals will understand this virus and other outbreaks going forward.

It is interesting to note that a Cleveland biotech company received approval at the end of March from the FDA to use stem cell treatment for bad pulmonary or lung problems that occur in coronavirus (COVID-19) patients. For the last five years in my practice I have treated emphysema and lung problems with intravenous stem cells. My results with patients have been good. This is a good move in the advance of medical treatment.

Preface

Healthy Life Reboot by Corbin Bosiljevac

In the springtime of 2020, outdoor activity across the nation was well underway, even considering the recently issued stay-at-home order. After months of cool weather, the enthusiasm for the season was not hampered by businesses closing or travel bans. We were nervous about the impending coronavirus yet still yearned to get outside and stretch our legs. Unique times like this help us to realize that our health greatly determines how dynamic and content we are as humans.

Americans crave happiness and a portion of this joy is dictated by the level of health each individual is living with. We are quickly realizing the benefits of a vigorous immune system and body. In a new age of medicine and the availability of drugs and supplements, we are often posed with the question, what is truly healthy for the body?

I have spent the last decade plus doing my own learning on the subject of healthy living. During this time, I began to think differently about my health and longevity of life.

First and foremost, I myself am not a doctor. Only my father is. However, I have had the privilege of being exposed to many forward-thinking health professionals. Some who are involved in stem cell procedures, others who specialize in immune boosting treatments, and more who concentrate on training amateur and professional athletes. It is their advice that I have grown to lean towards over the past 12 years and continue to employ in my own life practices.

In general, they view the body as a whole working machine. Instead of fitting an individual into a bracket or graph, they inquire about what level the body is functioning. When deficiencies arise such as soreness, immobility, or a diminished immune system (which is exposed during the breakout of a virus such as COVID-19) they take steps to locate the breakdowns. Just as a mechanic will perform a diagnostic check on your car to see what systems aren't functioning optimally, these cutting-edge doctors study where each individual is at, health wise.

The next step is to help individuals get to the core of the health problem and fix it. They take the time to get to know their patients and implore their best practices according to the individual's needs.

Finally, they recommend going forward that the patient have a more unique view of their personal health. Reboot the machine and then consider how to keep the body running at its ideal level. This includes eating, exercising and keeping the immune system in peak performance.

With this framework in mind, I yearned to stay active in life for as long as I could. Just because I had turned 40 didn't mean I should accept lower stamina, decreased mobility or lack of motivation. I had seen testosterone boosting commercials, but to me that seemed like a temporary fix. Getting the most out of life, and for as long as possible have become new goals to strive for.

So, I decided to be responsible for my own body, health, and lifestyle. I never wanted to depend on society to help me through my health problems. There was no reason to blame large food companies for my weight gain. Insurance companies don't have our best interests in mind and many commercials only want to suggest medicines that cover up problems but don't necessarily address the real issues within the human machine.

If I was experiencing discomfort or injury in life, I wanted to know how to manage this myself. The body is built for healing and I understood deep in my soul that we could live longer and more active lives if we took the steps to care for ourselves properly.

Following are a few odds and ends that offer how to begin to think differently about your health.

To understand what is truly healthy for the body, I consider everything that I expose myself to in the world. First is the food and drink I ingest. I use the mantra that I 'eat to live' as opposed to I 'live to eat.'

The things that I put into my body should be for performance reasons, fuel for life. I have learned that foods which are more natural, not processed or have a lot of preservatives, are better for me and my body performs more fluidly when consuming these.

When a person ingests unhealthy substances (which often taste incredibly good, unfortunately) it's as if he or she is poisoning him or herself very slowly. The effects are not noticed in mere weeks or months. Yet, over time the body's systems become tainted and the machine runs at a lesser level than it could be, therefore leaving the person feeling sluggish, sore, or unmotivated.

I always consider, 'how close to its source is this food that I am about to eat?' The body can digest and put to use substances that are clean much easier than 'dirty foods.' Processed sugars, fake foods, gluten, preservatives and starches are a drag to the body's natural system and the feeling of being tired and unenergetic are the byproducts.

Also, hydration is widely known as important to staying healthy and healed. There really should never be a reason to be under-hydrated in everyday life. Living in a first world country, we are privileged to have clean water at our disposal continuously. It is the vast access we have to sugary and caffeinated beverages that leaves us on the dry side.

One new practice is to take hydration to the next step. Consider where your H2O is coming from and see how best this liquid assimilates to your human machine. Water, just like foods, is often processed and the source and storage are hugely important in determining how healthy your water is. I suggest you do your own research on water sourcing and hydrogen tablets to help purify the body.

Next, I examine movement of the body. Activities for us to enjoy are at an all-time high. The evolution of sports, the availability of health clubs, and the ingenuity that we put into our individual exercise routines enable our bodies to last longer and to stay active well into our later years.

The key to staying fit at older ages is the type of workouts we do. After our prime ages from about 27-33, it is wise to adjust how we workout. Unless a person is training for a specific event, such as a marathon or maybe a mountain bike race expedition, then prolonged workouts aren't necessary.

For example, long jogs of several hours multiple times a week turn out to be detrimental to the hips, knees, and ankles as the body ages. Shorter workouts several times a week where the heart is increased to a high rate is more beneficial. I accomplish this by running at a high rate for 30 seconds to 1 minute and then resting for 1 minute before repeating. After doing this workout over the course of 10-20 minutes I feel great without having to indulge into an hours long commitment.

By all means, if you enjoy a long bike ride or jog then immerse yourself into what you love. The key is to realize that there are many means by which to get to the healthy end that you seek.

Going forward it's also important to do strength training several times a week, but also for only 20 minutes or so each session. This strength training keeps the body fit and able to support aging joints and limbs. Make sure you exercise both the upper and lower body but use lighter weight and do more reps.

Try applying a higher pace of work to this strength training to increase your heart rate. The idea is to get the heart racing higher than at a casual jog but for a shorter amount of time.

Strength training paired with your cardio work only needs to be in 10-40 minute intervals for 3-5 days a week. There should be a warm-up and cool-down period every time you engage in exercise. This leaves plenty of time during the week for the body to recuperate and ample time during the day to indulge in other activities. Your life doesn't have to center around exercise, but your mindset should center around healthy living in general.

Now, as with every workout it is important to keep the body limber through stretching, yoga, or pliability routines. I would suggest investing some time into becoming familiar with each of these in more detail. Just understand that these work together to keep the body feeling younger and more active throughout your years of life.

Natural immune boosting supplements are quickly becoming the most necessary addition a person can make to combat our changing environment. Elderberry extract, monolaurin, vitamin D, or multi-vitamins with Zinc are a great starting point. Going forward I plan to keep an eye out for information that educates me on ways to avoid a compromised immune system.

So, what is truly healthy for the body? We are in an era where information is easily accessible and the knowledge of how to preserve the human body increases every month. What was cutting edge a few years back is grocery store chatter these days.

What's important is to not be scared of thinking differently while you embrace change and enjoy longevity. Achieve this by consuming information and considering that the human body is a living machine that needs continual maintenance. The same old thing will get you the same old results.

I stand by a few statements that continue to hold true. Fad diets don't work for the endurance of life. As natural beings, we are meant to consume natural ingredients. And finally, where activity is important, so also is rest!

So, stay healthy and pursue in life what gets you to where you need to be.

The chapters that follow are timely and I spoke with my father numerous times over the initial days of quarantine around the nation. Our conversations centered around a changing American society, one that yearns to control its own destiny. Here we have learned that nature will tell you differently. Our destiny is already in place, and we are not the ones that know its fulfillment.

I hope this manuscript reveals enlightening material that will help you maintain your life in a nurturing path going forward.

Keep your eye out for my first book releasing later in 2021. It is titled "On to the Next Thing" and follows the imperative transformation of a man who spends 7 years in the Federal prison system. It is about growth, reflection, acceptance and forgiveness. We take in life what it gives us and if we play our cards right then we can move on in life, healthy and happy.

By the way, the man who spent those years in prison was me. Take control of those lifelong habits, get right, and move on to the next thing.

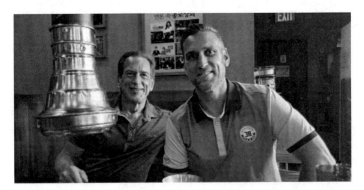

Joe and Corbin Bosiljevac enjoy a meal in Manhattan

I

Part One

Journaling through this Coronavirus Pandemic with regard to Health, Sanity, and How to Move Forward. With the onset of Stay-At-Home orders across the nation in March of 2020, uncertainty about personal health comes into question.

1

Hunkered Down on an Island in New York

19 March 2020

The coronavirus has us all staying and working at home as much as possible. The government and personal response have been good to decrease the incidence of the disease. It took a few days for the public to accept this but now subways and streets are almost empty.

We will learn more about the severity and contagiousness of this virus while waiting for it to mutate or change into a benign form. We will also learn how to more effectively handle this from a public as well as a medical standpoint.

Speaking of the medical aspect, there are early studies in China using stem cells and exosomes (growth factors) to treat coronavirus. Most deaths from the coronavirus are from respiratory origin such as pneumonia. Keep this concept in mind.

If stem cells are administered intravenously, they go to the right side of the heart and then are pumped out into the lungs. The stem cells get trapped in the capillaries of the lung. The lung is a perfect target organ for stem cell treatment. I have experience with stem cell treatments for patients with chronic obstructive pulmonary disease such as emphysema and some military who have been exposed to something in the air or environment causing chronic lung problems. Stem cell treatment has been quite successful to improve these conditions.

Many biologic factors contained inside a cell become depleted with age. The administration of exosomes and other biologically important substances can supply and increase some of these factors so the cell functions more optimally. Our system fights infections better.

Viruses are part of our environment. All of what is being done above is how we adapt for survival.

Oh, Happy Saint Joseph Day!!! March 19, 2020

Epicenter Report: Keys to Boosting the Immune System

22 March 2020

- We still need to follow the lifecycle of this virus, virulence, timeline involved, and its treatment to know more.
- Prevention with isolation is a big part right now.
- Personal hygiene measures and proper hand washing are necessary going forward.
- Pay attention to nutrition using a variety of whole foods - instead of packaged and preserved substances which do not promote good immune activity.
- Coconut oil contains lauric acid. When taken orally our bodies convert this to monolaurin. Monolaurin has a tremendous antiviral quality.
- It may be that antimalarial drugs like chloroquine will be helpful to blunt the viral response.
- Peptides that can boost the immune system can be used.

- Melatonin helps boost the immune system.
- Intravenous ozone has been used in the past with Ebola virus and was highly. effective. The big problem is having the logistics to be able to do this on many people at one time. But it is inexpensive, and it works.
- The use of stem cells and exosomes is a step forward in treatments. There is a good Chinese study demonstrating effectiveness with coronavirus. Basically, I look at this as boosting the immune system.
- This is a chance for us to grow together as a society. When was the last time the family stayed home together?
- Financially there are all sorts of consequences, short-term and long-term. It is a chance for everyone to reevaluate the importance of a healthy lifestyle.
- Can we handle this pandemic and learn to live together better as a society?

3

Corona Patient: How Difficult is the Diagnosis?

23 March 2020

New York City is overwhelmed right now with many coronavirus patients. Once screening tests are available, management of the infection may be more readily controlled. A big part now is social distancing and our understanding of health going forward.

I have a friend who is a 50-year-old black Dominican male. He is in good health with extremely low body fat. He eats a healthy whole food diet, takes supplements, and also uses alternative health methods such as red light and sauna. One of my observations was that it took 50,000 units of vitamin D per day just to get him into the upper normal blood level.

He became ill with no fever or gastrointestinal symptoms. He had no cough but just did not feel well. His wife is a registered nurse and she provides IV therapies for my patients. She keeps complete vital sign records on patients which includes measuring oxygen saturation. Now she checks her husband.

The oxygen saturation monitoring on his finger said 85% which is quite low and is significant to me as a doctor. Overnight it drifted down 82%. At rest he was not short of breath while not having any respiratory symptoms or cough.

He saw a physician in a 24-hour urgent care center and the doctor said there was nothing he could do for him and he should stay at home. That night his wife noted an oxygen saturation of 75%. Clinically, I am concerned at 85%, thus 75% is critical.

He presented to another urgent care center where the doctor looked him over and said he did not appear to have anything serious going on. An oxygen saturation was taken and it was 75%. Robert was sent immediately to the hospital where he later tested positive for coronavirus.

The key component here is that he didn't appear sick, but his oxygen saturation was dropping to near fatal levels.

He was in the hospital for about a week on oxygen. The CT scan of the chest was completely negative for any pneumonia or other abnormalities. Right now he just feels run down. His hemoglobin dropped from 13 to 9 because of lysis and destruction of red cells from the viral infection. Liver blood tests are elevated but this also is due to the viral infection and will resolve in 6 to 8 weeks. Oxygen saturation last night at home was 97%.

What occurred with Robert is medically noted as a cytokine reaction. He was very healthy and when this vicious virus hit he did not get violently sick. His underlying immune system fought and overcame it. However, the immune system kept going and overwhelmed him with a toxic hyper reaction.

He had a loss of taste and smell - many coronavirus patients have this symptom. With my surgical background I learned when patients reported this postoperatively that it was due to zinc deficiency. The symptoms respond many times within a week with additional zinc supplementation. My point here is that mild trace mineral deficiency, particularly zinc, may allow more susceptibility to viral infections. These are subtle things about our health that may be significant. Depleted cells can have these minerals restored as a part of a rebooting program.

Robert asked me with my judgment and experience if I could have made the diagnosis. My reply was no. With this pandemic, I told him, I did not want to see him. Just stay at home!!!! At this point in time we are ill-equipped to fight this virus head on.

Here in this link below is a more information on coronavirus resistance. I will be covering these more in detail throughout Part 2 of this book.

https://www.theguardian.com/world/2020/may/03/happy-hypoxia-unusual-coronavirus-effect-baffles-doctors

https://xkcd.com/2287/?fbclid=IwAR32j-So2lyuTH_cuP0Uu_PlZY quKdQ5ZRNg

4

What is it Like?

The season started with blossoms in the trees dangling moisture and smelling of warm concrete in the middle of the day. But the virus took away my time to visit Central Park. It snatched my chance for an extra walk around the block because the air smelled different than it does in January. For eight weeks during the spring there are different stages of foliage each year like a parade of flora. My apartment building has a circle driveway and there is a garden area with a fountain in front. I can enjoy the flowers there as well as beneath my fourth-floor balcony where there is a Bradford pear and two crabapple trees with hyacinths and tulips blooming. This is what it's like now, things in life were taken away so now I can rebuild with what is important.

It starts to get light by 5:30. Normally there are service vehicles and light traffic and I am accustomed to low continuous background noise after living in the city this long. Now it is noticeably quiet. I hear birds in the morning with their wake-up calls. Twittle-whirs and tweets-tweets. I don't recall these wonderful sounds. Before now it was rubber on concrete and shoes on pedals.

By **March 30th**, streets were not entirely empty, but a ninety-year-old driver could easily manage routes through Manhattan. I would say there was 1% of normal traffic. Now I can walk down the middle of 2nd Avenue in Manhattan for two blocks before I go back to the sidewalk because of traffic. A new adventure for me - Walking the empty streets in New York City. By **early April** pedestrian traffic was scarce.

Leaving my apartment to see an oral surgeon is the highlight of my social life right now. My Upper East Side apartment is only 4 blocks from my second office, so I walk there to pick up mail and deliveries before getting essentials at the local market. Upon my return home my hands are immediately washed. Shoes are taken off inside the entryway and slippers are used inside the apartment. This has been a regular practice for years. Now I also change clothes. The garments worn outside of my living space are put into the wash and I make my way to the bathroom for a shower. I figure this is the only way to be sure my world is not contaminated.

I do not have my dogs anymore or that would make it more difficult to manage cleanliness. My first seven years in the city I was known as the "man with three dogs." Here in Manhattan the only other people I recognized with multiple pets were the ones who owned businesses walking dogs or caring for pets. Mine are now all playing on a farm in Pennsylvania. Our time together helped me survive the move to New York and my divorce. Loneliness was not an issue with Bella, Mocha and Nanette.

Today there are many families cooped up together daily

and this is quite different for them. Outdoor activities are on pause right now. Some blocks within Manhattan may have 10,000 inhabitants and there is concern for spread of the virus because of the concentration of people. Everyone in our building has been gracious and within a week we just did not see anybody anymore. Not much coming or going. No jubilant salutations with the energy of a fresh season on the horizon. Just calm everywhere and waiting. Yes, the waiting.

When the USN Comfort hospital ship came to New York harbor on **March 30**, Samaritan's Purse began setting up hospital tents at 97th and 5th Ave. in the Central Park East Meadow. Across from Mount Sinai medical school I watch 250 ambulances that have been sent to the city by FEMA. More Ventilators are coming. The Javits Center has 1200 hospital beds ready, set up by the military after four days.

On the 30th I also took the subway. There was one other woman in the car wearing a mask and gloves. Phones typically are very dirty and are something that should be considered as far as personal hygiene. She continued to use her phone with her gloved hands but then managed to touch the face mask and scratch her neck several times. That is an example where the mask is not doing a lot of good for the person. I don't routinely use a mask but now that we are hitting the peak, I will do so anytime I go into a grocery store for essential shopping.

Wearing a mask could be a future standard for some businesses like a hair salon and barbershops as it may diminish the possibility of contact with other infectious diseases. The other thing to reinforce with people is good, frequent hand washing. To ride the subway and afterward get a cup of coffee and a donut without washing hands is not healthy. Hand to mouth. A mask certainly does help reinforce personal habits like Hand washing.

My girlfriend is from Korea and also has family in China. South Korea has reasonably well managed the coronavirus. As she pointed out to me, if the government there tells you to stay inside, then you stay inside. Orders as such are not as easily accepted here in the United States. We consider ourselves privileged and above recourse.

But the anxiety is an issue. Besides the risk of infection, the pandemic is currently creating economic challenges for many people. Suddenly life is more about survival.

Initially there was a stampede to all the stores for food and toilet paper. Other individuals show various degrees of anxiety. Consciously separating themselves on the sidewalk, I passed one who actually got off the sidewalk and walked in the street until I passed.

Even though grocery stores are empty there is concern about how many people have touched packages. In my apartment building some inhabitants do not want to get in the elevator with any other person.

My girlfriend lost her job. So many have and are uneasy because of it. She knows friends that have suffered from the outbreak in China. Now her current apprehension is doing Joe's laundry.

Everyone has been affected. Many people have lost work. The big anxiety for many is the economic catastrophe. I have high rent in Manhattan and yet the office is closed. I still spend time communicating with patients by emails and phone calls and began writing this journal to share health information. This does not bring in any direct income, but as a physician I would like to pass my experience on to patients.

This is about survival. We will all have challenges. One day at a time. Do what is right and step back to reevaluate. Then do the next right thing.

There are two stone lions outside the Manhattan Public Library. Below one is the word **PATIENCE**. Beneath the other it says **FORTITUDE**.

5

Alternative Treatment for Coronavirus

30 March 2020

From the epicenter: this pandemic is a big deal for our entire country. As I watch the US Naval Hospital ship enter New York City harbor today I am reminded of the military response to this situation. US citizens are used to seeing this on the evening news from across the seas rather than in our backyards.

There are further efforts with tents being set up in Central Park to serve as hospitals. Wound treatment during wartime helped develop many surgical techniques and healing principles. Now, the military has equipment and this is being used for peaceful purposes to help our nation recover.

There are several aspects for us to consider moving forward to improve health and prevent the spread of coronavirus.

1. The first would have to do with personal health habits.

- Here in New York, quarantine and personal isolation is essential. Many Americans are a little reluctant to have this imposition placed on their life.
- Families are spending the entire day at home together. This has psychosocial impacts because of the immediate and constant change this has placed on us.

2. The second area uses dietary measures.

- Ginger with echinacea and a little bit of raw honey may be helpful. Asians prepare this as a tea, drinking from 5 to 10 cups daily, although most Americans would not be compliant with that volume.
- Garlic taken orally has a tremendous antiviral effect.
- Coconut oil contains lauric acid which our bodies turn into monolaurin. This has a particularly good antiviral effect also. Monolaurin can be taken as a supplement or a tablespoon of coconut oil daily can provide good maintenance. This can be increased to three or 4 tablespoons a day if the patient develops symptoms.
- A lot of times dietary actions do not make a difference if done in a suboptimal fashion. To drink ginger tea may be accepted but to drink 10 cups a day may be difficult for most people to comply. However, dietary measures are a noticeably big deal as far as promoting personal health.

3. The third area regards ozone. This has been shown effective against the Ebola virus. Intravenous ozone is antimicrobial to everything. Conventional medicine and how to administer this to patients is not acquainted with

this procedure. However, ozone is very safe and effective. It is also dirt cheap.

4. Down the line a vaccination may be developed.

- The SARS viral infection occurred in 2003, it has been shown that this is a virus remarkably similar to the recent Coronavirus. As far as our normal immunity, exposure to something like that in the past may provide further resistance to this viral infection. In addition, patients that convalesce from the SARS viral infection may provide antibodies in their serum against coronavirus. This plasma can then be administered to actively infected patients, particularly those who are critically ill. If things are difficult to control, the use of SARS plasma could possibly be considered if there is a shortage of plasma from recovered coronavirus patients available.

5. One other thing to mention as lifestyle things settle down: consider doing a reboot of your cells and get your system running like it did 20 years ago.

https://www.linkedin.com/pulse/monolaurin-viral-infections-joseph-edward-bosiljevac-jr-md-phd-facs/?trackingId=2PYE70G4C

6

What is the Coronavirus Pandemic Teaching us about Health?

31 March 2020

- The recent coronavirus pandemic gives an opportunity to learn how to treat a new contagious viral disease as well as how best to control pandemics in general society.
- The coronavirus can cause pneumonia leading to a more severe illness and possible fatality.
- Stem cells show a significant improvement treating lung conditions.
- Plasma infusions donated by recovered patients can be helpful in severely infected patients.
- Exosomes provide another method of treatment for viral infections and rebooting cells.
- As a physician I follow a policy of good judgment and experience with the principle of do no harm.
- Despite lack of large clinical studies, use of treatments that may improve the condition with minimal risk can be considered.

• Patients benefit using medical judgment and experience.

The current coronavirus (COVID-19) pandemic is a major issue for the health of American people. Let me present some concepts regarding management of this infection.

In the human machine, good health is based on cells that are functioning optimally. Normal biologic factors that are present in the cell may become depleted with time or secondary to a disease process. Regeneration programs built on rebooting cells is the key since this leads to improved physiologic function. The cells work better. Rebooting is one aspect of wound healing which leads to increased ability to resist, recover, repair, and regenerate.

STEM CELL TREATMENT

Pneumonia and pulmonary dysfunction are the most frequent causes of death from the coronavirus. Patients with asthma, cigarette smokers, or those that have underlying heart disease are more susceptible to severe and fatal complications. As a physician my initial objective is do no harm. The second is listening to the patient, observe, and examine. This is how I develop judgment and experience.

I have a history treating lung problems with intravenous stem cell infusion. This includes patients with emphysema, asthma, and pulmonary fibrosis, all of whom responded well. Multiple groups have also shown similar results. I found out at the tail end of March that a biotech company from Cleveland received permission from the FDA to treat coronavirus patients with severe lung complications and pneumonia using stem cells. I have been using stem cells with lungs for five years and this makes me smile. Things are catching on.

CONVALESCENT PLASMA

There is a Chinese study with five patients treated using antiviral plasma from recovered coronavirus patients. This is another potential treatment which has been used before with other viral illnesses. Is convalescent serum from COVID-19 readily available?

Let us take this a step further. SAR S-Co -2 (involved in the six-month 2003 epidemic) is 95% similar to CoVid-19. How about treating patients with the available SARS antiviral plasma if the pandemic is getting out of control and supplies of corona plasma are unavailable.? The NHI and FDA require a lot of steps before treatments are approved. However, looking at the balance of risk and benefit, experience with other clinically potential options may be appropriate with a situation such as a pandemic. I say, let us be doctors.

It was announced recently that a program has been initiated to use infected corona plasma as a treatment. This relies on antibodies that have been produced by patients who have recovered from the viral infection. Early on there are mixed results. What are some of the gray areas or variables when trying to interpret clinical studies? Perhaps patients who do not respond well to the plasma have some sort of lazy metabolism and their cells are working sub optimal. It is very important to maintain optimal personal health.

EXOSOMES

Related to stem cells are exosomes, which are growth and biologic repair factors normally present in our system that encourage healing and regeneration. They decrease with age, can be rebooted with intravenous infusion, and may be combined with stem cell treatment or given by themselves. Exosomes have a tremendous anti- inflammatory property that improves immune system function and serves an antiviral effect. These biologic factors promote healing with nerves, brain, heart muscle, and provide wound healing and regeneration in many other areas.

EXPERIENCE

After 45 years in medical practice my judgment and experience help direct what is proper treatment for the patient. Stem cells, exosomes, and convalescent plasma are associated with little or no risk while the potential for benefit can be lifesaving.

It is difficult to initiate some of the personal measures mentioned above on a large-scale basis immediately, yet we learn with experience as we go through the current pandemic. There are essential personal health items that need to be addressed. Encouraging personal maintenance is essential going forward. Rebooting cells with normal biologic chemicals to function optimally. The human machine will then work better. Successful vaccinations will be available with time and perhaps released faster than other vaccines before.

https://www.linkedin.com/pulse/stem-cell-therapy-my-experience-optimal-results-joseph-edward/?trackingId=jSl7eFK8zz

https://www.ncbi.nlm.nih.gov/pmc/articles/PMC6739436/

https://jamanetwork.com/journals/jama/fullarticle/2763983

https://www.linkedin.com/pulse/benefit-rejuvenation-
joseph-edward-bosiljevac-jr-md-phd-facs/?trackingId=InaI4l78%2BLv

https://www.linkedin.com/pulse/exosomes-joseph-edward-
bosiljevac-jr-md-phd-facs/?trackingId=9qb9aFer%2F4sA9xspgGY%2F

https://www.linkedin.com/pulse/personal-maintenance-
reversibility-bosiljevac-jr-md-phd-facs/

7

Staying Home: What Occurs in the Mind During Quarantine?

4 April 2020

When you are bored, just think about a few things that don't make sense such as:

1. If poison expires, is it more poisonous or is it no longer poisonous?
2. Which letter is silent in the word Scent? The S or the C?
3. Do twins ever realize that one of them is unplanned?
4. Why is the letter W, in English, called double U? Shouldn't it be called double V?
5. Maybe oxygen is slowly killing you and It just takes 75-100 years to fully work.
6. Every time you clean something, you just make something else dirty.
7. The word 'swims' upside-down is still 'swims.'
8. 100 years ago everyone owned a horse and only the

rich had cars. Today everyone has cars and only the rich own horses.

9. Before biting a blueberry - what is the color inside?

8

Apartment Living

Personally, I am concerned about Florida, Louisiana, and Texas. Stay home. As I write this on **April 5, 2020,** *New York is at the apex as far as the daily new infection rate. The rest of the United States will be following New York City.*

This is not going to be about the cost of living in Manhattan although now I understand why it is higher here than living in the Midwest. I have a one-bedroom apartment in a building that was constructed in the 1960s. Rooms at that time were larger. What is not typical for a more recent one bedroom is that I have one full bath, one ½ bath and an extra room which may be a dining room. Instead I have made this my home office. My fourth-floor room has a balcony and when the weather's nice I am drawn outside to make phone calls, do paperwork, and watch New Yorkers scoot by.

It is **April 6th** and when I sit on the balcony there is no overhead traffic. None. Before I could identify four or five planes in the air at all times. Now there is no air travel. Growing up in the Midwest I have wilderness experience and recognize birds. I saw a bald eagle fly by close enough that it could easily be identified. There was nothing in the sky but the eagle migrating north. His life is the same.

The building in which I live has a doorman and a service area for deliveries. These days the doorman wears gloves and a mask while being very aware of the new standard health precautions. A self-service laundromat is open in the basement but I still have not spent any time down there. There is also a dry cleaner and laundry service inside the building. That part I do know - that's the one I use.

Daily emails are sent out by the building's management company that recommend how to maneuver within the current pandemic. Running this building is similar to managing a small town that rises high above the city streets.

I avoid elevators but that is no change for me since I am used to climbing the stairs to my apartment for exercise. To minimize personal contact the mailman has restricted access from apartment owners to mailboxes until he leaves.

The exercise room in the apartment building was closed on March 16th as per government recommendations. The gym is no problem for me since I have not used one for years and simply do body weight exercises after my stair climbing. I have a backpack that weighs about 30 pounds and will hike up and down the stairs with this. I am actually gaining a little more muscle mass because I am working out a bit more. Exercise is a part of the bottom line for helpful longevity.

With age many people back down on exercise. There are baseline low impact bodyweight exercises that can maintain good body composition and muscle mass exercising only 15 minutes four times a week. It is also important to do several minutes of intense exercise at least twice a week that help achieve a peak heart rate. I do this all without a gym and that includes when I travel. Although travel is not a good excuse for missing workouts, I hear this many times from my executive patients.

Here in Manhattan I am accustomed to taking shoes off and using slippers around the apartment. If I am on the subway I use gloves. Here in my apartment I will wash my hands as soon as I arrive and more frequently now.

My girlfriend is from Korea and also has family in China. She was working 15-16 hours a day in a restaurant and I would see her one day a week. Now the big change is that she is here daily. She keeps me informed on the viral endemic in Asia as she talks with her family. South Korea has reasonably well managed the coronavirus. As she pointed out to me, if the government there tells you to stay inside, you stay inside. That is not quite the acceptance here in the United States, even as it is one of the major points to control this pandemic.

The corona spread has caused some anxiety for her. She encourages me to wear a mask, but I refuse to do so when we are kissing.

With a 12-hour time difference from Asia she spends time in the morning as well as late in the evening to talk with family. My girlfriend spends the day cleaning, doing laundry (she doesn't want me to take my laundry to that laundry service across the street), and cooking whole food meals. She contacts friends to talk while I encourage her to learn and practice more English since she has more free time.

Immune system boosting will be important for many Americans going forward.

We follow a whole food diet. No processed food. No boxes, packages, cans, or bottled goods. Fresh, sliced, or pulverized ginger made into tea is helpful. Garlic has a tremendous antiviral effect. Add grated ginger and garlic together with some warm milk and honey. This does not taste bad and is extremely healthy.

Kimchi (fermented cabbage or radish) is another staple eaten daily and provides probiotic support. Eighty percent of the immune system is found in the gastrointestinal tract. The above are simple healthy lifestyle aspects that many times are lacking in American life. Add a little smile and an occasional hug.

Monolaurin can also be helpful. This is a derivative of coconut oil that has a tremendous antiviral effect. During this pandemic, a maintenance dose can be taken daily and can be increased to three or four times daily if symptoms and illness occur.

Peptides are bioactive proteins normally found in cells. Separate peptides can be used to support different biologic activities. TB 500 and thymosin Alpha-1 can stimulate the thymus gland and improve immune system function against corona and other viral infections.

I am sleeping a little later now and never watch television except for the news. Usually, I read books but now a few movies have crossed my path. One day all seven of the Star Wars movies were shown in series so I was able to reinvigorate the young man inside me.

I can answer emails and fill prescriptions and do other paperwork while the movie plays.

The government now tells us that this is just like staying home and watching TV all day. So pushing age 70, is this like retirement? Not bad. No responsibility to go to the office.

It enables me to write information related to the pandemic and share my medical experience and knowledge with patients. Except I have bills to pay. My girlfriend also has no work and has been sending money to her family. We are all in this together as a nation and will all learn and adjust our life. The bottom line is survival, it always has been.

At 7 PM every evening there is a lot of noise outside. The first time this happened I looked and could see people hanging out the window and waving. Everyone was blowing horns, clapping hands, and making all kinds of noise. This is just a neighborhood greeting that helps us all understand what we are going through together.

I open up the balcony and clap and wave. My girlfriend grabs my arm and pulls me inside when she thinks I am waving at the girl across the street.

Later I wander up to the roof. I can see the Empire State building from 35 floors up. Depending on the occasion or event, the Empire State building has many different types of light displays. On **April 1st**, it alternated with a combination of blinking red and white lights. This represents SOS. Other nights it will shine red, white, and blue - our nation!

9

Professional Life

When I moved to New York I started in an office on the 55th floor in the Trump building on Wall Street. The office was located a few blocks from the World Trade Center disaster, so I learned a lot about 9/11 and during the next 12 years much about the history of New York. I am a foreigner from the Midwest and the city's history is quite interesting to me.

For instance, in the mid1600s, the Dutch settled the tip of Manhattan Island. There were 'vicious' savages living to the north. A wall was built for protection and that is the origin of Wall Street. They also found out the Indians knew how to swim around it.

The Wall Street office is now closed during the pandemic, but the rent continues. For six years I worked at the Wall Street office on a daily basis. The last five years I only go down there about once every two weeks. The subway commute is only 30 to 45 minutes and the Q line leaves me 2 blocks from my apartment on 75th St.

I began to work in the Wall Street office a few years after 9/11. Although my exposure was remote, I have patients who lived and worked in New York City. They saw and experienced some of the consequences. They have shared with me their memories and feelings. The economic slowdown and closing of businesses during this pandemic will be much worse than what occurred with 9/11. Many people are dealing with fear of the future. One day at a time.

After developing a practice performing stem cell therapies, a second office space was subleased from a plastic surgeon. Lenox Hill Plastic Surgery is only four blocks from my apartment and turned into a wonderful convenience for me. So, I have two offices but the convenient one is my preference.

The view from the Wall Street office is super, but most patients prefer to see me at 79th St. For many it is more appropriate than driving into the business district down on Wall Street.

It has been a good experience with two offices in Manhattan. The plastic surgery office is robust with an operating room which provides me space to do stem cell procedures and injections. Dr. Rosenblatt, the doc who I work with there, does all of his surgeries in his office.

I have 12 years' experience with stem cell treatments. This includes patients with emphysema, asthma, and pulmonary fibrosis, all of whom have responded well.

Multiple groups have also shown similar results and I would consider the past 5 years successful in using stem cells with lungs.

Consider the anatomy and physiology of these treatments I speak of. An intravenous injection goes to the right side of the heart which pumps blood into the lungs. Stem cells injected intravenously will be trapped in the alveolar capillary membrane and initiate their repair of the lung from that area. Recall that I previously indicated pneumonia and lung complications as the main cause of death with coronavirus. ***Stem cells administered to a patient very ill with the coronavirus could help the pulmonary status.***

The first case reported was a 65-year-old female from Kunming treated with umbilical cord stem cells resulting in a remarkable recovery in two days.

Dr. Zhao from Shanghai University presented a small study including seven patients with favorable results using stem cells.

I found out at the **tail end of March** that a biotech company from Cleveland received permission from the FDA to treat coronavirus patients with severe lung complications and pneumonia using stem cells. I have been using stem cells with lungs for five years and this makes me smile. Things are catching on for medical treatment.

In **January**, before the concern of the pandemic, Dr. Rosenblatt told me that the office was being sold and I would need to find another space in the next six months. With the current pandemic it was directed in February that any elective medical treatment and surgical procedures be delayed until further notice. He may not be able to work for three months with the ban on elective surgery. The rent is high, and he told me to be looking for another office sooner than I expected.

Life is up in the air for many people. I see some professionals my age consider giving up their professional career. What a shame because of the accumulated judgment and experience of older, experienced doctors. From my standpoint I would like to mentor other doctors to be able to do some of the work with stem cells. I am too old to take care of a thousand patients. However, if I can mentor 10 doctors and they take care of a thousand patients each.

Two things have helped me considerably in my experience treating patients. The first is to do no harm. The second is listening to the patient. Observing, and examining is so beneficial and in my experience leads to better judgment.

My favorite mentor in my cardiovascular surgery residency was Dr. Jim. This was in the mid-70s and CT Scanners were just becoming available.

On early morning rounds before surgery we went down to the x-ray department to look at chest x-rays and a CAT scan. Afterward, walking down the hallway to make rounds Dr. Jim stopped and looked at me.

"Joe, if you spend the time listening to the patient and do the appropriate physical exam, 85 % of the time you will know the answer and do not need to do a CAT scan."

He turned and we continued our rounds. This is an example of good judgment from a surgeon who had a lot of experience. This is the same comfort level I strive to show each patient I interact with. God bless you, Dr. Jim!

Today, if you go to the emergency room with abdominal pain you get a CAT scan before someone even lays their hands on you or listens. The individual human machine is secondary to protocols and procedures.

Before I go back to the office, I plan to obtain a serology or blood test to see if I have corona antibodies. If I do, then this indicates exposure and resistance to this bug.

Looking for a new office I am focusing on some spaces within walking distance of my apartment. I have been spoiled with the luxury of proximity for years here in the city. However, for now I will stay at home and wait another two weeks before I even consider going out physically to look for a new space. Many physician offices are open for medical care with restricted hours, but elective procedures have been curtailed completely. In the meantime, several phone contacts have been made.

One of the office spaces available is with an older gastroenterologist who was Donald Trump's physician when the President lived here in New York City. It could be an unique adventure to work out of that office.

http://www.aginganddisease.org/article/0000/2152-5250/ad-0-0-216.shtml

10

Health Aspects

BASICS

For many years we have accepted flu virus epidemics. The coronavirus (COVID-19) pandemic was not expected. This virus has increased in virulence and has become very contagious. Viruses mutate and they can increase or weaken in strength.

I will not review a lot of science regarding viruses - this is readily available in various medical and news reports. I continue to follow medical reports here as well as other countries. It is difficult to know whether someone is a carrier. Only about one in a 1000 people will become infected. Of those that become infected about 2 in 100 will die.

The most important initial requirement for prevention is social distancing and staying at home. Personal hygiene aspects are especially important. Increased availability of screening tests and serology to check for protective antibodies will be helpful long-term in the control of this pandemic. I plan to obtain a serology test before I go back to work in the office.

The next aspect is looking at the federal and state government response to provide supplies for treatment and other medical care. The military serves a tremendous role to help the entire country. Samaritan's Purse set up the Central Park East Meadow field hospitals across 5th Avenue from Mount Sinai Medical Center. Another field hospital was opened up at the Billie Jean King tennis center.

We can be grateful for continued increased voluntary and corporate support. I see us helping each other. The importance of responsibility for personal and lifestyle changes can improve health and encourage resistance to further pandemics.

From the lifestyle standpoint, social distancing is the most important measure. Churches, schools, nonessential stores, restaurants, and bars have all been closed.

People are encouraged to stay home and work from there when possible.

The most frequent symptoms with coronavirus are fever, sore throat, gastrointestinal symptoms, and cough. Heart and lung complications from pneumonia are the primary fatal symptoms.

The case study presented was associated with a cytokine reaction, which is simply a hyper reaction from the immune response of the patient.

One of the subtle signs is redness around the eyes. This is not redness in the white part of the eyeball but in the skin around the eye socket.

Another interesting sign is loss of taste and smell. In my surgical career I would occasionally see patients for a postoperative visit and they would mention loss of taste and smell. This indicates a relative zinc deficiency that will respond to supplemental zinc while symptoms can abate within a week or two. Zinc has certainly been shown to be beneficial in preventing upper respiratory infections and is involved in wound healing.

How is this related to coronavirus? I notice that many times trace mineral deficiencies may not make the patient sick enough to go to the emergency room. This is very subtle. However, it may mean that the overall human machine may not be functioning properly with decreased immune function ability. 'Reboot your system' is what this says to me.

There is a relationship involving a ratio of zinc and copper together. Copper is an important element that is also involved with the function of the immune system.

Trace mineral deficiencies may be affecting overall metabolism - perhaps in a very subtle way. Lack of certain trace minerals may also affect intracellular hydration. I am not convinced that current medical reference ranges are optimal including recommendations for supplemental intake.

An important aspect with trace minerals is that they may be absent from plants or produce because of depletion in the surrounding environment. The appropriate food is eaten, but the nutritional value is suboptimal.

On **April 6th** it was reported that convalescent coronavirus serum was being used in seriously ill patients with mixed results. Suboptimal cell function from nutritional as well as other elements can play a part as far as the overall treatment outcome. Less healthy patients do not survive.

There are ways to evaluate and follow levels of minerals using an oligoscan. This bedside exam uses an infrared light to look at about 20 different trace minerals and additionally a dozen toxic heavy metals. It uses tissue levels (not a blood or urine test).

The exam is accurate and consistent when followed in a serial fashion and can monitor if supplements or other treatments are being effective. The oligoscan exam collects objective data on mineral balance and can help direct measures to balance the overall human machine and improve wound healing.

Now look at some basics regarding wound healing and health.

Light is extremely important (I'm talking about sunlight not indoor artificial lights). Lights inside a room do not emit some of the wavelengths provided by the sun that stimulate normal biologic activity. Ultraviolet radiation from the sun kills viruses. Infrared wavelength stimulates nitric oxide production in our bodies for healing.

Another thing to consider is the blue light from any device like a computer or television screen. This can alter the circadian rhythm and balance of various hormones. This is more important with the computer or your phone since these are close to your face.

Plus, more people are spending considerable time in front of the computer screen. The use of a blue light filter, which can be a pair of special glasses conveniently kept at the side of the computer, may also play a part here.

Why discuss 5G technology during this pandemic? Electromagnetic waves can subtly disrupt our resistance by interfering with the biologic function of our cells.

Be aware and consider this when looking at overall health in the long run after the pandemic. My concern is recent research implicating that 5G can cause mutation of viruses to a more virulent form. This can be a big factor for future epidemics. Biologic activity can be affected by an electromagnetic component.

An important aspect of wound healing and health is water. Most processed water has had a breakdown in the geometric symmetry of the water molecules. Water is a liquid crystal just like glass. When the crystalline structure is broken down the water is not assimilated into the cell as easily. This structure can deteriorate inside a plastic bottle.

Processed water is also likely to be deficient in trace minerals. Chronic intracellular dehydration does not necessarily mean a dry mouth or feeling thirsty. This is an example of a subtle aspect of health - cells that are dehydrated do not function properly.

The emphasis here should be rebooting cells to restore normal biologic agents that deplete with age. Rebooting cells. An overhaul rather than just an oil change.

When we are talking about epidemics, it is important to encourage optimal personal health in the community. This not only involves treating an infection but also prevention. The healthier the individual the less likely to have a severe infection. Some recommendations about personal health can be addressed in the future after this pandemic.

Nutrition is a big part of overall health and some other aspects will be discussed next. Current treatments that are possible with stem cells, exosomes, and plasma infusions will be covered later.

https://www.dailymail.co.uk/health/article-8148851/Nurse-says-red-eyes-telltale-sign-coronavirus-infection.html

https://www.linkedin.com/pulse/5-g-technology-safe-joseph-edward-bosiljevac-jr-md-phd-facs/?trackingId=OhgKdVsPU4C

https://www.linkedin.com/pulse/hydrogen-water-joseph-edward-bosiljevac-jr-md-phd-facs/?trackingId=hoYvgr9Lw1%2FX9Xg

https://www.linkedin.com/pulse/personal-maintenance-reversibility-bosiljevac-jr-md-phd-facs/

https://www.linkedin.com/pulse/what-does-mean-reboot-joseph-edward-bosiljevac-jr-md-phd-facs/

11

Early Stage Developments

Mid-February I was down for two days with a fever and a sore throat. Five days after the fever left, I finally felt back to normal.

My younger son came to visit me on **March 5**. During that trip there were no restrictions and life was typical New York City. He has not been ill through today.

Coronavirus (COVID-19) began in Wuhan province in China. There were some deaths and reports indicated this was at the level of a severe flu virus. It started back in December and progressed into January. During that time there was a lot of travel between China (Chinese New Year) and the United States. New York City has a large Asian population and is a primary entry point for travel.

I have been undergoing oral surgery and was in the middle of a three-part procedure that started early March. On a follow-up visit back on **March 9** the subway was about 75% full. I was careful to wear gloves while traveling. The oral surgeon took my temperature and checked me over before the procedure was started.

Around **March 10**, the government was encouraging social distancing. Churches were locked up and schools closed. My impression is that this was not taken very seriously by New Yorkers for about a week or so since there was crowding in the parks and children were out playing on the sidewalk without proper social distancing. It was like one big spring break outside similar to the disregard given by spring breakers in Florida.

Nonessential stores closed including restaurants and bars, although delivery or pickup was available at the restaurants and bars during restricted hours. By **March 16** there began to be a reduction of activity outside when the city closed many parks and basketball courts. I live one block from the subway and I noted there was only about 50% of the normal activity with much work being done from home.

Supermarkets stay open but for caution have limited entrance. Service was provided early in the morning for elderly persons and those handicapped. (Hey, I am a senior citizen). Afterwards, a line would form outside the supermarket for the rest of the day. The line had people 6 feet apart for social distancing. Five people are allowed in the store every so often as the store empties. There are a lot of people that live here. At least most are not going hungry. Food is present but the street side produce sellers and sidewalk cook carts are gone. So much for a quick hot dog or soda.

I returned to the oral surgeon on the **23rd of March** and individual pedestrian activity on the outside was 20% normal. This included traffic. If I wanted to get a taxi it would have been difficult but not entirely impossible.

Another appointment was on the **30th of March**. At this

time the subway was only about 10% full. Grand Central Station normally contains thousands of customers by late morning but was essentially empty. The subway back to my apartment had two subway cars completely empty with each third car containing one or two persons.

On **April 1st,** the U.S.N. Comfort hospital ship entered New York Harbor. At that time, it was taking non-COVID patients in an attempt to relieve pressure from other medical emergencies affecting the hospitals that handle infected patients.

By the **first few days of April**, Mayor de Blasio was recommending everyone wear masks outside. When I go on the sidewalk and there are no other pedestrians I may leave my face open. My two-part plan inside a grocery store is to first put on a mask or scarf. Secondly, I hold my breath as long as I can. Well it's a one-part plan anyway because part two is hard to do for more than a minute or two. The overall idea is to promote people to think healthy.

Nail spas finally closed and then so did the barbershops. Boy, do I need a haircut! I timed that one poorly, but it helps save money. And I can take some hippie photos in about a month of my long hair—and this is with no grey hair at age 70.

Essential services remain open and this includes the laundry and liquor stores. Maintenance needs to be provided for the apartments and other buildings. Buses and subways continue to run, although not as frequent. Garbage and recyclable collection as well as service such as propane delivery continue.

I heard from a colleague that Milan has been using drones to decontaminate public spaces. Is this what is next for us here?

On **April 6th,** the evidence may be beginning to show if appropriate social distancing measures are taken that it takes about two and half weeks for instance levels to begin to drop. That is where we are in New York City today. In Italy and Spain it took over four weeks, but they started the social distancing much later.

On **April 8th** I went to Staples today to buy ink. It was a pleasurable walk of 12 blocks and I encountered only one other pedestrian each block. Over half of the people I encounter are wearing face masks. Traffic is about 5% of its usual. Staples has plastic shields for protection for the cashiers.

On the **16th of April** I took the subway to the oral surgery office. The subway was about 20% full, which meant we were able to sit down with two to three spaces between us. Some were wearing masks. I wore gloves and it was easy to practice social distancing in the subway car. There were still considerable vehicles driving on the street although these primarily consisted of delivery and service trucks. Nonessential medical services and surgeries have been canceled for probably the next two or three months. Some medical offices are open for other health care with restricted hours.

Instructions from the media and the government were to restrict activity to home except for essential items such as groceries. Medically, they were looking for more masks, gloves, and protective coverings for hospital workers. New York was seeking a large number of ventilators. Some dentists, plastic surgeons, anesthesiologists, and veterinarians have ventilators in their offices. I have one about 35 years old that was used during my former practice, but I do not think they will want to use that unit.

When I first moved to New York I owned a car, so I have experience driving in Manhattan. Usually I would park long-term in a parking garage. However, sometimes if I were using the car for errands or to take the dogs to hike in Harriman State Park (I had three dogs in Manhattan for seven years), I would try to park the car outside the apartment on the street. This cannot be done forever because street cleanings are scheduled two days a week. Cars need to be moved and there is a large fine or the vehicle would be towed. Well, I sometimes got a break when there would be a holiday and I could leave my car parked outside for almost a week. Usually it's only two or three days working around the system of street cleaning. **Alternate side parking restriction has been postponed until April 20.** Park your car and leave it until that time without moving it! If it is used to run an errand the same parking spot may still be open later when the task is complete. No one is driving. This is another unique and original occurrence for New York City. 9/11 did not do this.

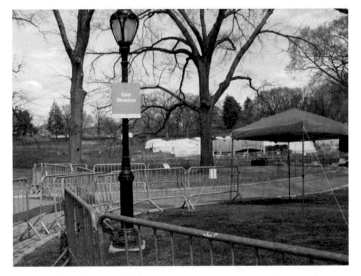

Samaritan's Purse field hospital in Central Park.

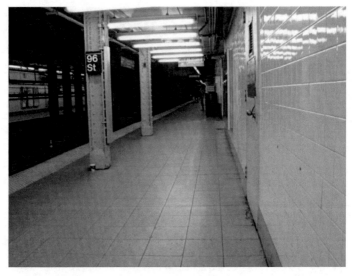

Subway at 96th a few weeks into the stay-at-home order.

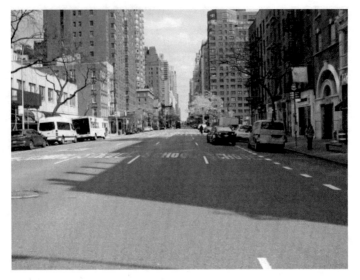

3rd Avenue and 75th on April 1st.

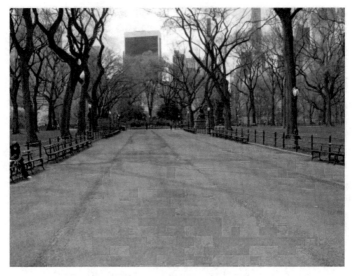

The walk into Central Park on April 1st.

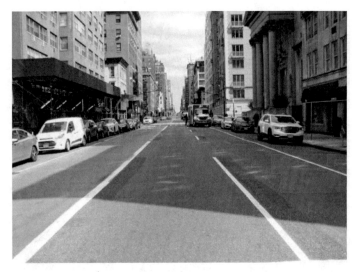

Lexington Avenue on April 1st.

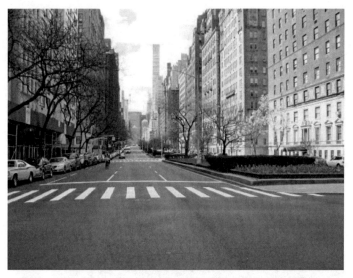

The view down Park Avenue during the start of the stay-at-home order.

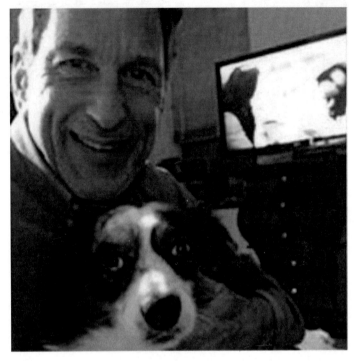

**Nanette (Australian Shepherd) and Joe ready for a
Central Park tour.**

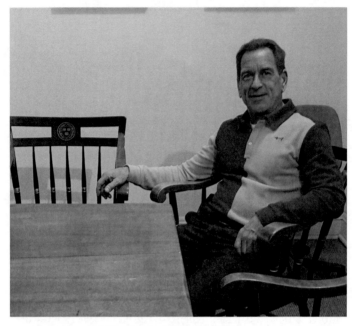

Doc Joe pushing 70, before a holiday party in 2019.

12

British Healthcare Workers Press Release

16 April 2020

Late in 2019 with the onset of the COVID-19, a study was set up using Povidone Iodine (PVP-1 - or Betadine for us Americans) for a nasal spray and mouthwash during instances of high contamination.

PVP-1 is a good general disinfectant and has good antiviral qualities. It can be applied to mucous membranes inside the nose or mouth, which is where the virus collects. Viral content was measured in healthcare providers as well as patients during the general hospital care for COVID patients. Mucous samples for virus were taken frequently when there was exposure to the oropharyngeal tract such as intubation.

First of all, it is safe for the nose and mouth with proper dilution. Exposure to iodine during this study was well within previously recorded safe levels.

Second, it significantly reduces the viral load on surfaces where droplets from sneezing and touching the mouth are encountered.

Third, it was shown the effect can last for three hours.

Get a nasal spray of normal saline (0.9% sodium chloride) from the pharmacy. Use half the contents of this bottle and add the same volume of the standard Betadine solution. That is your dilution. As mentioned, it appears an application lasts for three hours. It can be sprayed into the nasal passages as well as the mouth. As far as the mouth application, wait one minute or so before any water or other things are ingested afterward.

This is another example of something learned from experience with this pandemic. The use of a Betadine type spray in the nose and mouth is so effective, convenient, and inexpensive. A simple way to Improve hygiene as part of our lifestyle.

13

Corona Survival

19 April 2020

After a month, most people here in Manhattan are accustomed to a daily home routine. I am apartment bound, answering emails and doing phone calls with my patients. In a few instances I will do a Skype consultation. One of my offices is four blocks away. I'll venture down that way with a mask and gloves every other day for faxes and mail. Masks are compulsory at this time. There is a scheduled complete shutdown until May 15 Today is Sunday. I took a nice slow walk today.

Pedestrian traffic is about 25% of normal and street traffic is about 5%. People are quite cautious including only one person or couple using an elevator at the same time.

The 7 PM neighborhood salute is beginning to lose enthusiasm after a month. Another thing that I see is less socialization and conversation with people wearing a mask - not even saying hello or good morning.

I am the sole proprietor in my medical office with a high

overhead. No help from SBA. I am not the only one in this situation. Office and retail space in Manhattan are quite expensive. Many other people have been affected economically with sudden job loss. There is a prediction that one out of three businesses will close permanently following this pandemic. That is much worse than the effects of 9/11 on New York City.

Testing is the key right now. A recent report out of Santa Barbara, California where testing was done on a large number of people suggested that perhaps 50% of persons were carrying Corona antibodies. This is a good start. I'm using an FDA approved test that is also being used by the United States government for their employees and military as testing increases.

If you have positive antibodies you are protected. Get back to work. If not, another game plan needs to be approached as far as getting back to work in a normal society. The sample of tests arrive midweek and I will do this on myself and report at that time. You will hear controversy regarding whether this antibody is long-standing. If I were your physician and your antibody test was positive, I would be comfortable with you having a normal lifestyle and recheck you in six months.

22 April 2020

10 o'clock and no one is out on the street. Traffic is maybe 20% of normal with cool spring weather present all around me. Trees are blooming and fortunately there are several around my apartment. My testing kits for antibodies arrive at the office today. One of my offices is located four blocks from my apartment. I can easily get there for mail and

deliveries. The office is closed, but I can schedule private appointments with patients for antibody testing.

14

Ozone / Oxygen Therapy for Coronavirus

Many surgical techniques and knowledge of surgical care and wound healing came from the battlegrounds. As a clinician you learn from experience while this pandemic is another opportunity.

During my career I have taken care of many patients on a ventilator. Early planning with the pandemic led to the accumulation of these. Ventilators help people breathe better and were felt to be an urgent aspect to battle the coronavirus since serious respiratory or lung problems can occur. 80% of corona patients that are on a ventilator do not survive.

The patient needs more oxygen. Clinicians want the oxygen saturation of blood to increase. Breathing oxygen through the nose is not enough. Oxygen can be administered for breathing but it is not getting into the blood. There is a thickening of tissue from the inner lining of the lung that impedes diffusion of oxygen into the blood vessels of the lung. Oxygen just cannot get into the blood. Despite a ventilator, oxygen is still not getting in. Finally, the patient expires.

The patient needs more oxygen. So, clinicians consider other methods since the ventilator does not appear to be the key to treatment of lung problems.

Can oxygen be infused directly into the blood? You cannot do this with oxygen, but you can with ozone. Oxygen in blood increases, cells function more optimally which can enable the patient to recover. IV administration of ozone is a short-term method to get over the hump. Clinicians really appreciate a quick field goal. I have used this treatment in my practice.

The Spanish medical force has used ozone administered through the vein with success.

This is inexpensive and effective. Just like a battleground we continue to learn. Further in this writing will present in more detail this ozone approach.

Ozone in an instant:

- Ozone is a highly reactive form of oxygen.
- Ozone contains 3 rather than 2 oxygen molecules.
- Ozone in the upper atmosphere is protective of our environment.
- Ozone combines with industrial emissions to form SMOG.
- It has potent antimicrobial properties and can be used in the treatment of acute and chronic viral illnesses.

Ozone is a highly energized form of oxygen found in nature. It consists of three oxygen atoms bonded together where oxygen primarily exists as two atoms. Ozone presents as a molecule with a third oxygen atom that is highly reactive and wants to leave the group. This provides the oxidant quality of ozone that can be used for our own health benefits. An oxidizer is different from a free radical. Oxidants are not bad - they help us get rid of the "junk" that resides in our bodies. Ozone already has many industrial applications because of this characteristic. Dave Asprey explains the health benefits of ozone.

Ozone forms in the atmosphere as the effect of ultraviolet rays from the sun. It can also form after an intense electrical charge, such as lightning. Sometimes the faint smell of ozone can be detected after an intense thunderstorm. I even smelled ozone in the air once following the flash of a large meteorite.

Once ozone forms in the upper atmosphere it can protect us from the longer wavelength ultraviolet B radiation - this is the type that can penetrate our skin causing sunburn.

Chlorofluorocarbons are ozone depleting chemicals that have reduced this protective ozone layer. Ground-level ozone is formed by burning fossil fuels (hydrocarbons).

Although it can detoxify cyanide and help urea decompose, it is considered a pollutant when combined with industrial emissions. High levels of smog can cause scratchy, watery eyes and respiratory symptoms. Ozone can be encountered indoors around electronic equipment and photocopiers. Could this perhaps be related to many people's "allergy" symptoms?

As a powerful oxidizer it can serve an antibacterial purpose in municipal water systems. The antimicrobial property (as well as that of hydrogen peroxide) can be used in food preparation. It affects organic molecules so it can be used to remove pesticides from fruits and vegetables. How about as an alternative to chlorine to disinfect hot tubs?

Now, how is it used to fight viruses?

White blood cells secrete hydrogen peroxide as a way to fight microbes that cause infection. Ozone destroys the fatty outer cell membrane of microorganisms. Viruses that contain many lipids (fats) in the cell membrane are very susceptible. Ozone therapy can be used for severe acute viral illnesses. Look at what Dr. Frank Shellenberger stated in 2014 during the Ebola virus:

"Just to recap, about four weeks ago, I reported that past Second Opinion editor Robert Rowen, MD had teamed up with Dr. Howard Robins to bring ozone therapy to West Africa. Why? It's because ozone therapy has been successful in treating every viral Infection we have ever tried it on from hepatitis C virus to West Nile virus to herpes virus — all of them. So it made complete sense to think that it might also be an effective treatment for Ebola virus. But was it to be?

"Just before the treatments were about to be given, a phone call came in from the health ministry telling the doctor in charge, "If you want to keep your job, you will not permit any ozone treatments in the center." I'll leave you to conclude why this sudden change of face. I'll leave it to you to ponder why a safe, inexpensive therapy with a successful track record for viral infections was forbidden to a group of patients the majority of whom were sure to die. I'll leave it to you to connect the dots. How could it happen that the health ministry, which was the only collection of high level officials that did not attend the trainings, could possibly find a reason to forbid any safe, inexpensive, oh, and yes, unpatentable and unprofitable therapy to be given to these dying patients?"

Ozone therapy can also be used in the face of chronic viral illnesses such as HIV, Epstein-Barr, cytomegalovirus (chronic fatigue syndrome), and chronic hepatitis C. I have seen patients with chronic symptoms from these conditions, as well as Lyme, improve with treatment.

Here is a reference to an article that came out on **April 14th** that shows Spain joining other nations using non-pharmaceutical drugs successfully with COVID-19 patients. Patients who were failing with oxygen levels and were about to be intubated were given intravenous ozone. Repeated ozone treatments diminished the rate of intubation 80% because oxygen saturation improved following the ozone treatments.

Ozone is improving oxygenation at the cellular level while cells are being rebooted in this example.

The First Patient:

A 49-year-old man who had already required ICU admission was deteriorating on the ward. He had deteriorated to the point that he required oxygen at the highest concentration and yet it was oxygenating his lungs poorly. Intubation and connection to a ventilator was planned, but surprisingly, after the first session of Ozone therapy, the improvement was significant and oxygen requirements could be decreased.

Dr. Alberto Hernández explained that:

"The improvement after the first session of Ozone treatment was spectacular. We were surprised, his respiratory rate nor-malised, his oxygen levels increased, and we were able to stop supplying him with as much oxygen since the patient was able to oxygenate himself.

To our surprise, when we carried out an analytical control, we observed how Ferritin, an analysis determination that is being used as a prognostic marker in this disease, not only had not followed the upward trend, but had decreased significantly; that decline continued in the following days. This result encouraged us to administer it to other patients who are following the same improvement as our first patient."

Ferritin (a blood test) was mentioned above, and this is part of my routine blood work when monitoring patients. It is an excellent marker for inflammation when elevated. It also correlates with recovery from the disease or condition when it decreases. That is a nice fact to know as additional data to help manage someone that is severely ill such as with the coronavirus.

This pandemic - and I live in the epicenter in Manhattan - allows an opportunity to see and feel the experience of this illness. What I publish about the coronavirus epidemic here in NYC is already past time. The ballgame continues to be played with further decisions pending. This may open up "out of the box" and non traditional lines-of-thinking for many people as far as treatment options.

https://blog.daveasprey.com/ozone-therapy-benefits-safety/?mc_cid=c7b6b7025e&mc_eid=4ac2791235

https://healthimpactnews.com/2020/after-seeing-great-success-spain-approves-ozone-therapy-for-covid19-patients/

15

Treatment Advances with Coronavirus

TODAY'S REVELATIONS:

- Lung problems are the most common fatal complication.
- Stem cells have shown to provide effective treatment.
- Dr. Joe can do Zoom.

The concerns about virulence and fatality with the current pandemic can lead to some significant changes in medical care. The availability of surveillance testing is limited but this will change. This is important since vaccinations may not be available for 12 to 18 months. Patients want to get back to work.

I have kits available to do a blood test in the office looking for Corona antibodies. For me, that is the basic test. In 10 minutes I can tell you whether you are positive or not. If you have antibodies there is nothing to worry about. If the antibody test is negative then I

will do a nose swab to see if you are carrying this little varmint.

The big deal with the coronavirus is related to the lung. Originally thought to be a type of pneumonia, the process actually displays aspects of physiologic changes similar to what occurs with severe high-altitude sickness.

In that condition the inner lining of the lung will become swollen with fluid so the transmission of oxygen from the lung into the blood is markedly diminished.

As mentioned previously, I have more than five years' experience giving stem cells and exosomes to patients for lung problems with success. Multiple groups have also shown similar results.

Look at the anatomy and physiology. An intravenous injection goes to the right side of the heart which pumps blood into the lungs. Stem cells injected intravenously will be trapped in the alveolar capillary membrane and initiate their repair of the lung from that area. Recall that I previously indicated pneumonia and lung complications as the main cause of death with coronavirus.

Stem cells administered to a patient very ill with the coronavirus could help the pulmonary status.

The first case reported was a 65-year-old female from Kunming treated with umbilical cord stem cells resulting in a remarkable recovery in two days.

Dr. Zhao from Shanghai University presented a small study including seven patients with favorable results using stem cells.

There was a recent report out of the Jerusalem Post describing complete cure from coronavirus in five patients treated with umbilical cord stem cells from the Israeli company Pluristem.

The Israeli report demonstrates 100% survival rate. The stem cells help regenerate damaged tissue as well as provide an anti-inflammatory effect. These cells regulate T-cells and M2 macrophages which cause inflammation. This is similar to what I have seen in my practice, particularly with autoimmune cases.

There is a lot of discussion and controversy on the use of stem cells in medical practice. The FDA is easing restrictions as far as introducing this into the care of Corona patients that have severe respiratory problems. I can assure you, this technique is scientifically sound and has been effective in my practice for patients with chronic lung problems.

This may become an accepted practice more quickly than what may have happened without this pandemic.

Another area that can be approached would be rebooting cells. When cells have appropriate amounts of all biologic factors they function more optimally. This is the key.

If you have a patient who is ill and a rejuvenation program is used to reboot cells, many symptoms will abate. Then you can have a more focused program to direct further recovery for patients.

Now, I am an old man pushing 70. Recently, I have been doing more Skype interviews in my practice, particularly with new patients since I cannot see them in the office. This technology is going to push us to another level of care in standard practice. Old men must also learn…or get older and dumber.

https://www.webmd.com/lung/news/20200407/doctors-puzzle-over-covid19-lung-problems?ecd=wnl_spr_040720&ct

spr-040720_nsl-LeadModule_title&mb=lGVdiurmHBMQOzQuk

https://www.linkedin.com/pulse/corona-patient-how-
difficult-diagnosis-bosiljevac-jr-md-phd-facs/

https://www.ncbi.nlm.nih.gov/pmc/articles/PMC6739436/

https://www.mystemcelltherapy.com/2020/03/coronavirus-
critically-ill-chinese-patient-saved-by-stem-cell-therapy-
study-says/

https://www.jpost.com/HEALTH-SCIENCE/Israeli-
COVID-19-treatment-shows-100-percent-survival-rate-
preliminary-data-624058

16

Nutrition

Nutritional aspects of general health and specific areas related to coronavirus have some early and long-term benefits.

When thinking about food the first step is the whole food concept. Sometimes when I suggest to patients not to carry any boxes, cans, packages, or bottles from the grocery store they comment "Gee, then I would not have any groceries." Processed food may not be recognized by the stomach as beneficial nutrition and includes exposure to chemicals and preservatives.

Also look at items such as maturity of the produce. Fresh foods that are picked too soon may result in diminished vitamins, trace minerals, and other nutritional elements. In addition, produce to be shipped is sprayed or processed to maintain a fresh appearance.

In his recent book called Plant Paradox, Dr. Gundry cites a statement from the FDA that the "nutritional aspect of our current growing environment is depleted or very nearly depleted at this time." Most nutrition books talk about food and the associated vitamin and **mineral content, which may be much lower than anticipated depending on the source** of the product. Dr. Gundry points out the importance of **source**, something not commonly covered in many nutrition books.

Grass fed beef is entirely different from corn fed. This is the same for dairy products. Farm raised fish is not the same as wild fish. Again, we are talking about additives, preservatives, hormones, and antibiotics that are used with the animal during growth. Dr. Gundry also points out that the FDA statement above is from 1936. Where are we today?

Think about the source when considering what vitamin and mineral supplements are contained within what you ingest. Depending on the characteristics of growing or raising a food product, there may be lack of trace minerals and other nutrients. So, two apples from different sources may not be the same, and I am not talking about the taste.

When I practiced in the Midwest many of my patients were ranchers. I was offered the opportunity to hike their land when looking for deer antlers with my dogs. I found this rejuvenating to spend time in nature and rewarding to see my dogs run in the open fields.

Out one day, I saw Dr. Browning, the owner of the Browning ranch for pasture raised cattle and/or also a practicing physician in Kansas. I walked out to say hello and to see how the season had been treating him.

He explained that there is an Asian plant called Lespedeza and that one of the species is a vining type plant. These can be seen in the southern states hanging from overpasses on the interstate. Bill had recently sprayed because this plant was growing in the pasture. The cattle that roamed this same land ate the grass that had been sprayed. So here is another variable I will throw out at you:

Even though the beef is grass fed, can it also be contaminated with insecticides, herbicides, and other chemicals? Be aware of these aspects and then simply just do the best you can.

If patients follow a good whole food diet 5 to 6 days per week, they do not need to take a multivitamin daily. Also, it may not be necessary to take certain supplements every day. Patients with iron deficient anemia taking an iron supplement on an every other day schedule actually assimilate and increase iron levels much quicker than taking this on a daily basis. It may not be necessary to take a lot of supplements daily. And as a final thought, think in terms of the source and preparation of the supplement to be used. These are items that make a difference whether the product is good quality or not.

Conventional medicine continues to accumulate more hard data in evaluating trace mineral deficiencies. Suboptimal levels do not bring on any acute symptoms where the patient winds up in the emergency room. So, there is no urgency. I am not convinced that the current reference ranges and recommendations for mineral intake is optimal.

With this most recent pandemic, I would like to first introduce aspects related to improve general health and then apply this to the coronavirus. An example would be zinc.

Many coronavirus patients suffer the symptoms of both loss of taste and smell. With my surgical background I learned when patients reported this postoperatively that it was due to zinc deficiency. The symptoms respond many times within a week with additional zinc supplementation. My point here is that a mild trace mineral deficiency, particularly zinc, may allow more susceptibility to viral infections. These are subtle things about our health that may be significant. Depleted cells can have these minerals restored as a part of a rebooting program. Zinc and copper ratio is important with overall health. Copper is important with many enzyme activities and heart muscle health. It helps protect the immune system and keeps hair from getting gray.

A whole food diet with appropriate nutrients and trace minerals is about 80 to 85% of our health. It is important to keep cells healthy. An individual can reboot cells by restoring healthy biochemicals to the cells so they function optimally.

Adequate hydration and optimal trace mineral supplementation need to be considered as building blocks.

To repair, restore, and regenerate is rejuvenating the human organism.

17

Smoked

When I first noted an outbreak of coronavirus in Milan as well as Spain, I felt that this may be due to the fact that there is a higher population of smokers in these countries. The attached article demonstrates that cigarette smokers are one fourth as likely to develop coronavirus. This is interesting since the most severe complications of coronavirus are related to the lungs. Could nicotine be doing this? Or is this just the toxic smoke killing the virus? Just an observation as I attempt to learn more from this current pandemic.

French researchers to give nicotine patches to Coronavirus patients and frontline workers after lower rates of infection were found among smokers:

- A French study found that only 4.4% of 350 coronavirus patients hospitalized were regular smokers and 5.3% of 130 homebound patients smoked.
- This pales in comparison with at least 25% of the French

population that smokes.

- Researchers theorized nicotine could prevent the virus from infecting cells or that nicotine was preventing the immune system from overreacting to the virus.
- To test this theory, hospitalized coronavirus patients, intensive care patients and frontline workers were given nicotine patches.

https://www.dailymail.co.uk/health/article-8246939/French-researchers-plan-nicotine-patches-coronavirus-patients-frontline-workers.html

https://www.dailymail.co.uk/news/article-8264635/More-proof-smokers-risk-catching-coronavirus-expert-admits-weird.html

18

Blacks and Corona

Statistics have shown that black patients have a higher mortality rate with coronavirus and these numbers are consistent here New York City. The majority of blacks have incredibly low vitamin D3 levels. I am not singling out a particular race strictly on statistics. I have also noted lower vitamin D levels in black patients during my career.

This is my line of thinking after understanding the benefits of vitamin D levels over my last 20 years of immune boosting work.

Vitamin D has a chemical structure similar to that of a steroid like testosterone and estrogen. I tend to consider it a hormone. Cholesterol is a precursor which forms vitamin D.

Here are the variables. When vitamin D or sex hormone levels are suboptimal, cholesterol goes up. When vitamin D levels are restored, cholesterol comes down without medication. I have seen this time and time again. An individual with a more active lifestyle and good vitamin D levels has healthy natural sex hormones without taking supplements.

The **normal reference range** for vitamin D with conventional medicine is **30 to 80**. Most blacks have levels below 30, and some black patients of mine have required 20,000-50,000 units of vitamin D3 daily just to achieve a level of 50 or so. Many of my white patients take 5,000 to 10,000 international units daily to get to a level of 80. Not only is it interesting to see the different doses that are required for a positive response, but it may indicate that the reference range is not completely optimal.

What I do in patient care is learned from experience with thousands of patients. Following treatment with stem cells, If I have 20 out of 25 patients with an excellent result and there is no clinical study supporting this, I can honestly and professionally use my clinical judgment as far as treating individual patients. Good judgement comes from experience and follows the principle of **First do no harm**.

Vitamin D provides a tremendous **anti-inflammatory effect**. Pushing doses to the range of 100 with patients that have a lot of soft tissue aches and pains is helpful. Vitamin D has an incredibly good anti-inflammatory response and has been shown to improve recovery when fighting viral infections. High levels of vitamin D also improve sugar metabolism in patients with type II diabetes. I have yet to see any toxicity the past 20 years even with patient vitamin D3 levels of 110 to 120. I am not sure the reference ranges are optimal.

Many patients will tell me they do not take vitamin D because they are outside in the summer sun. Sodium benzoate, a common food preservative, as well as other chemicals can actually interfere with the conversion of the

D2 form to active D3. Many of these patients who are in the sun still have low vitamin D levels. This may be in the 30 to 40 range, which is accepted by conventional medicine, but is this an optimal level for that individual?

Clinical studies attempting to confirm the medical benefits of vitamin D can be associated with other variables that affect the result of the findings. Sometimes these variables are not considered as part of the clinical study, yet they may influence the results. This includes lifestyle variables such as diet, smoking, alcohol, obesity, exercise levels, and others.

We are going through a learning phase with the coronavirus. Perhaps the increased incidence and mortality in blacks with Coronavirus infection *may* be associated with *suboptimal* vitamin D levels. So, there may be a short-term response acutely with coronavirus patients, but also long-term benefit to balance the immune system using vitamin D. And I have seen no toxicity with this routine.

It is best to take the vitamin D3 at bedtime. In 80% of patients this initiates a better sleep cycle. Cortisol levels drop and growth hormone can increase naturally with better sleep.

I have had patients troubled with seasonal affective disorder (SAD). If their usual dose is 10,000 units of vitamin D, they are told to double that dose after Labor Day and continue until New Year's Day. 20,000 units daily of vitamin D3. This has helped relieve symptoms in many patients with this condition.

https://www.wsj.com/articles/vitamin-d-and-coronavirus-dispari

https://www.linkedin.com/pulse/unique-aspects-vitamin-
d-joseph-edward-bosiljevac-jr-md-phd-facs/?trackingId=Yl87UiYq9V

19

Dogs vs. Corona

A recent news story indicates that dogs are being trained to detect Coronavirus. Similarly, there are reports in the past where dogs were used to detect cancer. For example in my reference below, Rosco does bedbugs.

My brother, who has security experience, expanded that this can be used at the admission entrance when there is a large event. The use of a security dog in buildings with a high activity level like a shopping center, grocery store, or movie theater may be helpful. It is reported that up to 750 persons per hour can be screened.

Take it one step further. Public areas frequented by many people can be assessed by a dog while the space is empty to see if there may be a deposit of viral contaminant. This can then be cleaned. We can look at potential carriers, but the dogs also present a way to expeditiously clean activity areas.

Part of learning with this challenge is to be open-minded and to think of health as preventative and not reactive.

https://www.mirror.co.uk/news/uk-news/coronavirus-dogs-being-trained-diagnose-21885979

20

Can it Come Back?

21 April 2020

Here in the epicenter of New York City, recent daily statistics show that cases of hospitalization as well as deaths may be slowly declining. It appears that we have reached the peak and hope the incidence will continue to decrease. There is a question as to whether any antibodies to the coronavirus formed at this time would be effective if there is a recurrence of the disease in the fall.

Corona viruses (there are several types) are **enveloped** RNA viruses. This means they have a solid outer protective layer. They come from a series of viruses that typically have symptoms similar to the common cold. Two strains, severe acute respiratory syndrome coronavirus (SARS-COV) and the Middle East respiratory syndrome coronavirus (MERS-COV) cause severe respiratory or lung symptoms. Both of these and all the coronavirus are zoonotic - which simply means they can be transmitted between other animals and man.

So here are the next steps:

1. Testing is a big step at this point in the recovery in New York City.

2. These tests need to be done in a professional manner to maximize accurate data.

3. **The test that I use has been accepted by the FDA** and is also being used by the United States government for their employees as well as military personnel.

4. Testing will give statistics as far as overall incidence. A large sample of testing done in Santa Barbara California suggested positive antibodies may be found in up to 50% of the general population.

5. I hear criticisms about the validity of serology or blood testing. This is typical testing done for Epstein-Barr virus (EBV), cytomegalovirus (CMV), and many others including coronavirus.

6. If antibodies are present, is the patient protected from another outbreak in the fall? Antibodies confer the ability to fight infection after exposure. If antibodies are present, the patient is protected from the infection at this time. Whether this expands to resistance in the fall for this coronavirus, I cannot give you an answer. As far as human survival and resistance, positive antibodies can usually protect for a significant time during an epidemic. How long does that last? Experience will tell us. Accept that you are protected but continue to follow personal hygiene.

7. If the patient is antibody positive, they can go to work and not worry about excessive protection. However, self-hygiene items such as frequent hand washing is still recommended.

8. If the patient is antibody negative, I will do a nasal swab

and then repeat this after two or three days. This will confirm if the patient is an asymptomatic carrier. It will also direct the ability to get back to work in general society.

9. An antiviral, non-pharmaceutical treatment plan can be recommended for patients with negative antibodies. This may include monolaurin, zinc, and vitamin D.

There is concern that coronavirus can mutate into less or more formidable forms. This is part of the concern for outbreak in the fall. Many factors can affect mutation of viruses. One of the very subtle variables can be 4G and 5G technology. These have been shown to possibly introduce mutations in viruses. Think outside the box for long-term survival.

https://www.linkedin.com/pulse/monolaurin-viral-infections-joseph-edward-bosiljevac-jr-md-phd-facs/

21

Closing April

24 April 2020

Today is rainy. It has been cool with temperature peaking in the mid-50s for the past 10 days. Warmer weather and sunlight can help overcome the virus.

I am tired of the apartment and actually losing track of which day of the week it is. It helps to make up a daily agenda. There is just no urgency.

I make trips to the office for mail every other day. Very few people are going out and there may be two people out walking in one block. When people are wearing a mask, they are not talkative despite attempts to be friendly. Street traffic is 20% to normal.

The evening 7 PM neighborhood get-together is not as exciting. Nobody has any new type of noisemaker.

At least my apartment building has a garden area outside with trees that are blooming, tulips, the burning bush. These and other things that make spring better.

25 April 2020

Today is comfortable to sit on the balcony with the jacket while reading and writing. I left my phone off and ignored it all day.

I pour a Johnny Walker Blue for a toast. One month out. It is nice being outside today. I will go to the rooftop later where there are several trees and a very nice view.

The 7 PM neighborhood salute was loud! Everyone is celebrating Saturday.

26 April 2020

Same old same old. It is raining all day. The 7 PM neighborhood salute was quiet. I do not have a DVD player. Called my kids while watching movies. Reading books.

27 April 2020

New York City is still not quite over the crest of the epidemic. The newest release is that China found an antacid drug, famotidine, that may have assisted in recovery in some patients. I do not think recovery will be as easy as a drug cure. Clinical studies attempting to confirm the medical benefits can be associated with other variables that affect the result of the findings. Sometimes these are not considered as part of the study, yet they may influence the results. This includes lifestyle variables such as diet, smoking, alcohol, obesity, diabetes, exercise levels, and others.

22

Testing

Surgical techniques and wound care principles were learned from battlefield conflict. We now have a war with the coronavirus presenting another chance to learn something beneficial. Stem cell treatments may be a resource offered to patients, but for the next six months I will be a Corona Doctor in NYC. This is not my usual practice, but to provide testing and guidance for patients the next few months is part of age management and survival.

Coronavirus Testing

- Can it come back?
- Can I get it again?
- What does it tell me?

Concern with the recent coronavirus is the danger of reinfection. A vaccination may becoming but none for SARS nor MERS (cousins of coronavirus) has yet to be developed.

This is a new zoonotic virus (zoonotic - occurs and can transfer between animals and humans) and this pandemic is the first contact with a human. It is unknown if it follows the course of previous viral infections.

Let us look at the sequence of a virus infection. The patient has what is called a **first response,** which is generally non-specific and involves fever and other common symptoms. This is the body's manner to try and resolve the infection. The virus is killed because of active T lymphocyte cells. Antibodies (Ab) are formed for protection. The presence of B lymphocyte cells serve as memory to produce an antibody if there is another encounter with the virus.

The infectious course may be:

1. A few viral particles cause an asymptomatic infection, but no antibodies are formed - *the body is strong enough to resist.*
2. Asymptomatic infection occurs with antibodies. **The patient does not carry the virus and is not susceptible to infection.**
3. A symptomatic infection occurs with positive antibodies. The patient **does not carry the virus** and is not susceptible to infection.
4. A symptomatic infection occurs with no antibodies formed (which can occur in 30% of the infected patients). This may be part of **a suboptimal healing response**.

In Iceland, 50% of the general population are asymptomatic Ab carriers of coronavirus. The tolerance with this pandemic may be due to genetics. Improved nutrient and mineral density of food and animal products, and the use of high-quality animal protein in the diet may lead to a high level of resistance.

Different populations may have had an asymptomatic disease and developed antibodies (ranging from 20 to 50%). Think about the difference between white versus Asian, for example.

Patients may have such a potent immune system that it overcomes exposure to the virus but is not enough to produce antibodies in their bloodstream. Maybe B lymphocyte cells are not working properly. It may also represent the individual is immunocompromised or this represents a delayed individual response to develop antibodies.

There is suboptimal immune function overall. Only 70% of convalescent patients have developed antibodies. Recovered patients can be a source for convalescent serum but not everyone can be a positive donor of convalescent serum.

My guidelines are the following:

1. Give the serum antibody test for IgM as well as IgG. If IgG is present, then no restrictions are necessary.
2. If a patient is IgM positive and IgG negative, it indicates that they are early in the course of the exposure. In this case, I would do a throat swab and then repeat the blood test for antibodies in two or three months.
3. **Remember 'hygiene best practices' in all cases**.
4. If serum antibodies are negative, a nasal swab test will be done to see if the patient is an asymptomatic carrier.
5. Caution needs to be taken as far as social distancing if there is danger of infection.
6. I will also recommend several protective measures:

- Availability of KN95 medical mask for protection.
- Look at betadine saltwater nasal and throat spray. This

is convenient, effective, and inexpensive.
- Monolaurin 3000 mg a day as a maintenance dose.
- Repeat testing for antibodies in three months.

These are my concerns:

1. Vaccinations have not been developed for SARS and MERS, both of which are cousins of the coronavirus. Those outbreaks are now controlled because large portions of the population are naturally immunized. That, in essence, is what vaccinations attempt to do - they may not be a good option here. Time will tell.
2. This virus is zoonotic so there may be some unknowns that we will not foresee. However, this will also help teach more how to manage epidemics in the future.
3. Improved hygiene and nutrition measures in the population are part of our survival.

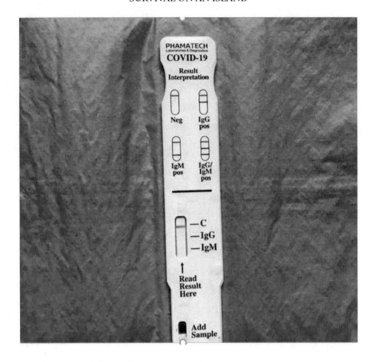

Well, I got mine and you can see in the photograph the results. When the C line lights that means the test technically was done properly. The other areas to look at are the IgG and IgM. If lines occur in those areas, it means you have been exposed to or currently are recovering from the coronavirus.

So how do I interpret this? First of all, I have never been exposed and my body was not pushed to make any antibodies. I will begin to see patients in the office, screening them for return to work and daily society. I will be following usual protective measures in my personal contact with patients. I will be using the antibody test first of all. If the antibody test is negative before they go back to work, a throat test will also be done. In addition, I have an itinerary for patients to use if they still need protection.

Among these:

1. The NP 95 protection mask (medical grade mask) when needed for high risk areas.
2. The use of monolaurin as an antiviral protection agent.
3. Repeat testing can be done down the line in follow-up.
4. Remember good personal hygiene in all cases.
5. Vaccination when available.

23

An Ounce of Prevention vs. A Pound of Cure

On April 22, 2020 During a phone consultation with a Panamanian patient, I asked about the status of corona in his country. He said there were some cases, but everyone was isolating themselves. The rule in Panama City was three days a week only men could be out doing errands. Three days a week only women could be out doing errands. On Sundays no one is allowed out.

Foods, Vitamins, and Supplements during the Pandemic

Testing is coming. No vaccination has been produced at this point. The best measures in today's battle with the coronavirus are personal hygiene as well as eating a wholesome diet.

Viruses are part of our world and will never be eliminated. Many references cover nutritional aspects of foods. There are supplements that contain substances that fight infection, such as Echinacea.

Rather than a complete review, I refer you to other sources available. My clinical goal is to develop a program that is convenient as well as manageable for each individual person. Some basic background will be presented on a handful of foods that can be used on a daily basis for an antiviral effect.

It is important to note qualities of trace minerals. Zinc can help with upper airway sources of viral infection since it protects the mucous membrane lining of the nose and throat where the virus attaches. Many coronavirus patients have a loss of taste and smell.

With my surgical background I learned when patients reported this postoperatively that it may represent a relative zinc deficiency. The symptoms respond many times within a week using additional zinc supplementation. My point here is that mild trace mineral deficiency, particularly zinc, may allow more susceptibility to viral infections. Depleted cells can have these minerals restored as a part of a rebooting program.

Trace minerals serve an important part in many biologic activities. Trace elements and minerals can have a complex relationship with each other. Zinc has a relationship with copper which also boosts the immune system. Significant biologic changes can be affected. Symptoms of deficiency may be so subtle that no one needs to go to the emergency room.

Trace mineral deficiencies can also affect intracellular hydration. Minerals work with water as far as balance, effective movement inside and outside of cells. I am not convinced that current medical reference ranges are optimal including recommendations for supplemental intake. Trace minerals may be depleted or absent from plants or produce because of depletion in the surrounding environment. The appropriate food is eaten, but the nutritional value is suboptimal.

Grass fed beef is entirely different from corn fed. Same for dairy products. Farm raised fish is not the same as wild fish. Again, we are talking about additives, preservatives, hormones, and antibiotics that are used with the animal during growth.

There are ways to initially evaluate and follow levels of minerals using an oligoscan. This office or bedside exam uses an infrared light to look at levels of about 20 different trace minerals and additionally a dozen heavy metals. It measures tissue levels (not a blood or urine test). The exam is accurate and consistent when followed in a serial fashion. The oligoscan collects objective data on mineral balance to assess whether supplements or other treatments are being effective for optimal balance and improved overall healing of the human machine.

The oligoscan can also look at heavy metals. Cadmium, mercury, and lead can adversely affect the immune system. There are good heavy metals such as iodine and selenium. With low tissue iodine levels, the function of the thyroid gland may be variable so that it is better one day than another. Persistence of symptoms of a low immune system can be a subtle sign of trace metal deficiency or heavy metal excess. Although these may affect an acute illness, these aspects may be more important regarding long-term prevention.

Garlic has tremendous antiviral qualities. I became more impressed with this herb root while working in a third world country. A doctor there asked me about the US practice if someone had an upset stomach. I told him an endoscopy (to look inside the stomach with a scope) and then probably prescribe some medication. The doctor told me that they had no scope available and patients could not afford medication. He told me that adding ginger and garlic to their diet not only has an antiviral effect, but the garlic actually kills helicobacter pylori, which is a bacteria that commonly causes stomach problems. This is part of the environment they have lived in for generations.

After the onset of the virus, my Korean girlfriend fixed up a concoction that had garlic and vodka together. This does not taste good. I do not recommend this. It is still sitting and will continue to do so. If something is bad, as it gets old does it become less or more bad?

Cumin seeds have a specific anti-inflammatory activity that improves digestive complaints. Affecting the G.I. tract helps stimulate the immune system, most of which is situated around the intestine. Turmeric and black pepper also have an anti-inflammatory effect.

Ginger is another spice with a tremendous benefit for the stomach. Improving the ability of the stomach to empty results in acid reflux symptoms that go away. Just like that, Prilosec is gone. The antiviral use of ginger is to drink tea two times a day. For an antiviral effect when symptoms occur, it may be necessary to drink five or six 8-ounce glasses of ginger tea daily. So, part of the recovery depends on acceptance from the patient for a mode of treatment done in a manageable fashion. Do they get it done? Compliance, that is the patient's part.

Ginger also has an anti-inflammatory property and can be used frequently with cooking. My girlfriend took another step (as is with our extra time in the apartment) and prepared a drink that contains ground, steamed ginger and garlic, honey, and warm milk with turmeric and cinnamon. Really not too bad! And it is healthy because of its rebooting qualities.

Ginger can also be used in bone soup as it restores growth factors and other biologic proteins that encourage repair and regeneration. This was a staple for my grandmother and mother and is standard for Korean and other Asian people. This is part of a whole food diet. Slowly boil the bones overnight, adding garlic, onions, and vegetables including ginger. The bone marrow releases growth factors. This is a good method with acute illness as well as once every three months just for rebooting. My grandmother prepared it once a month.

Vinegar is also effective for antimicrobial properties. A small amount of apple cider vinegar with the diet is helpful. Vinegar is quite useful in general as a decontaminant for the room - avoiding chemicals.

Monolaurin and Viral Infections

Coronavirus and other viruses are part of our world and will never be eliminated. They can potentially mutate and become less or more virulent. That is a method for their survival. Our survival is resistance or repair and recovery after exposure to these guys.

The Human Machine needs to be ready to HEAL.

A natural and highly successful preventive measure involves the use of coconut oil. Coconut oil contains lauric acid and our body converts this to monolaurin, which has an antiviral quality. I had one patient with HIV who had high viral loads. These dropped down considerably after using monolaurin and no other change in his treatment. I saw the same in a patient who had chronic active hepatitis C.

So monolaurin is not specific, but it has a tremendous overall antiviral effect. The optimum dose for daily maintenance is 3000 mg. This can be increased to three or four times a day with the onset of any symptoms. If monolaurin is not available, two tablespoons of coconut oil daily is a good maintenance dose. This can then be increased if some sort of infectious symptoms develop.

Surgical techniques and wound care principles were learned from battlefield conflict. We now have a war with the coronavirus presenting another chance to learn something beneficial.

Stem cell treatments may be a resource offered to patients, but for the next six months I will be a Corona Doctor in NYC. This is not my usual practice, but to provide testing and guidance for patients during the next few months is part of age management and survival, so this is right in my wheelhouse.

Healing and caring for the human machine are of utmost importance, it always has been. It has taken drastic changes in everyday life and now in our financial climate to get society's attention. The good thing is that we are learning from this new situation, and quickly are able to turn our experience into knowledge. Now, my hope is that our knowledge continues into action.

https://www.linkedin.com/pulse/what-does-mean-reboot-joseph-edward-bosiljevac-jr-md-phd-facs/

24

How to Survive on an Island by Corbin Bosiljevac

The way I see it, this is only the beginning of an adventure. Right now, most middle-class New Yorkers are struggling to survive economically. Like other events in history such as 9/11 or Pearl Harbor there is life before these events and the lifestyle after. Manhattanites state that this is worse than what occurred with 9/11.

We are vulnerable as human beings, but we are not vulnerable as a human race. When our collective consciousness evolves in a harmonious way, we thrive together.

Begin to view your health not just as a way to appear well to others, but as a way to prepare yourself for the onslaught of life. Nobody else will take your well being seriously unless you do, and then it is an ongoing march. Live and continue preparing yourself every day for it. This knowledge here is only armor to keep you vibrant throughout your years of life. **Survival.**

As this adventure develops, we will see the outcome of the pandemic within the NYC epicenter. Medically, we will learn. Social and lifestyle changes will also occur. This is a challenge to become better. Continue reading as we journal through this pandemic towards recovery and our new age of health.

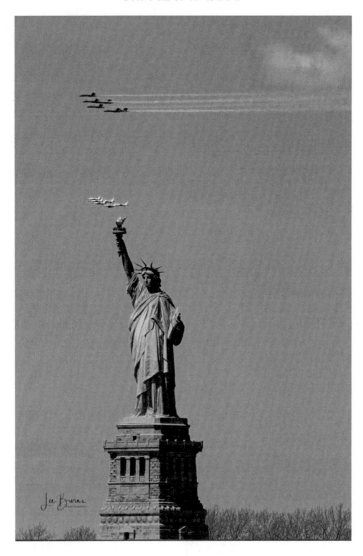

II

Part Two

Coronavirus Pandemic - Resistance and Recovery

25

As it Sets In

In part 1 we discussed how coronavirus was initiated by the sudden onset of quarantine and health regulations that changed and advanced each progressive week. Information was flying before us by the second and I used this time to reflect, observe, and conclude that our personal health on this planet is going to be of utmost importance moving forward.

Our race has seen struggle, and experienced triumph and strife in the past, but as with anything that is new, the anxiety was high. The main difference with this new pandemic was the government control of the economy and its directive into how we should deal with our personal well-being. Our health seemed to NOT be in our own hands, and it was frustrating. Many times, people do not recognize they also have to be responsible. So, I strived to bring peace with some advice for the situation going forward.

Part II will look at recovery and resistance. Aspects as far as short and long-term lifestyle changes that improve resistance will be presented. This entails medical advice that most anyone can involve into everyday life. I have dealt with medical situations my whole professional career and just as so many other professions, change is certain. Some of this material is never offered to patients through conventional medicine. This is not some new sensational health advice, but it does speak to personal discipline and an open-minded approach to health.

So goes my advice partnered with my personal journal through this time. I felt it important to show my human side during this unique experience while offering my judgement for all of us to consider when it comes to personal health. In the chapters that follow we can observe where the world stands at this point in history.

BENEFIT FROM REJUVENATION

It seems obvious to me and I'm still not sure why more health professionals are not discussing this with the general public. I suppose the reasons come down to convenience, money and effort. It takes a unique lifestyle to value health and time over assets and income, but that is what I am offering. Instead of talking to you about investing money into your retirement account, I suggest you invest effort into your longevity. This is where I highlight the benefits of rejuvenation.

I spent 29 years in a solo practice doing cardiovascular surgery near Kansas City. I have also obtained a doctorate in natural medicine, giving me a very wide background and experience with over 45 years in both conventional as well as alternative medical practices. During my surgical career I operated or helped operate on every part of the body. As a surgeon I was involved with the post-op healing process. Principles learned as a surgeon regarding wound healing are a basic part of my practice including stem cell treatment.

The rejuvenation program that I present to patients is a process of <u>rebooting cells</u> to function optimally. When the body functions well at the cellular level, then the whole organism is more fluid in its efforts. This is done by replacing or restoring proteins, growth factors, enzymes, and other biologic substances that are used by cells for function and regeneration.

A. If you are 50 years of age, understand that many of the biologic chemicals in our cells have diminished or become depleted. Much of this happens in a very subtle way. You do not have to go to the emergency room or necessarily feel 'sick.' Society accepts that 'you are just getting older.' However, rejuvenation is possible. We do not have to become immobile just because we are getting older.

B. In cases of chronic disease with multiple symptoms, there may be innumerable visits and treatments from many subspecialists. This can be extreme and time consuming. A process of rebooting can eliminate many of the symptoms. After rejuvenation, a simpler and more straightforward program for further recovery can be presented to these patients. They can fire half the doctors. They are better because the cells are functioning better. I consider this an overhaul rather than oil change. Regenerative therapy is boosted by using principles of wound healing.

Practicing age management in New York City the last 12

years, I quickly found that getting older means body parts wear out. Working with retired NFL and NBA players I began doing stem cell treatment for joint and soft tissue injuries. Then I started treating military Special Forces members. With this group I began dealing with other conditions such as traumatic brain injury, MS, emphysema, autoimmune disorders, and liver problems as well as regeneration from various soft tissue and joint injuries.

Biohacking is my game plan. From my surgical background, this is all a matter of wound healing. Agents used in this treatment course are part of normal biologic substances that are present, but depleted, in our system. The first step is optimization of the patient's chemical and hormone status and can be done to promote regeneration and healing. Light and oxygen are also used as part of stem cell treatment. Interval reappraisal of the patient directs further recommendations for regeneration of tissue. This is where various peptides have come into play as part of the overall picture.

BPC 157 is one of the most frequently used. The military guys and retired professional players have been beat up all over. General uses of this peptide for soft tissue and joint problems have certainly been extremely helpful. If the patient has a specific joint issue or a tendonitis such as tennis elbow, they can be instructed to give the injection around any bothersome area. There is a high initial local tissue concentration before the peptide is absorbed systemically. This can rapidly improve results over an acute or chronically diseased area. I have seen this clear tennis elbow pain within two weeks. A peptide such as BPC 157 is usually used short-term for 1 to 3 months. This is basically giving fertilizer to the human machine to repair. This has been my experience.

An interesting note is that BPC 157 is a peptide of gastrointestinal origin. Many chronic gastrointestinal complaints like acid reflux and irritable bowel symptoms disappear within a couple of weeks after initiating this peptide. I have seen in most patients a definite gastrointestinal benefit despite giving the peptide for another reason.

REBOOTING THE NAVY SEAL

Here is an example of a special operations patient:

There is a 58-year-old Navy SEAL who was seen three months after his "brain quit." His history revealed multiple concussions which include a fall from rock climbing and multiple blast injuries. He was institutionalized and started on hyperbaric oxygen treatment, showing some improvement after 20 treatments. Overall, his mental clarity and focus were blunted and he had bilateral tinnitus and intermittent dizziness. Speech was sluggish and at times a little slurred. He had degenerative condition of both knees and his low back due to years of packing a lot of weight while on deployment as well as parachute drops. He had left sacroiliac impingement as a component of the back pain.

He had a partial left knee replacement and about a month post op this was hyperextended stepping down. The left quadriceps at the distal femoral attachment was painful. There was pain in the left shoulder with tenderness over the biceps insertion but maintained full range of motion with the shoulder itself. The patient also has a history of chronic acid peptic disease.

Understand, all portions of the program are to re-boot cells and improve metabolism to what it was 25 years ago.

The first part is to initiate chemical and hormone optimization. The patient was started on bioidentical testosterone which promotes rehabilitation and rebuilding with wound healing.

Following this, the patient had two days of intravenous NAD (nicotinamide adenosine dinucleotide) infusions. Recall that diseased and affected nerve tissue dumps out NAD. Then neuropathies develop.

During the NAD infusion there was improvement of the tinnitus as well as the speech. *I have many MS patients who had significant improvement in neurologic symptoms with NAD given intravenously. This is only temporary—you are filling up the NAD gas tank. However, it also indicates that stem cell therapy can give long-standing benefit. When patients improve dramatically with the IV infusion of NAD, I am confident they will respond favorably with stem cells given in a wound healing environment.*

On the third day intravenous exosomes (growth factors) and umbilical cord stem cells were infused systemically. This was done using wound healing adjuncts such as infrared lasers to stimulate nitric oxide production and hyper oxygenation. I also performed an exosome injection into the distal left quadriceps.

Finally, the patient was started on the peptide BPC 157 as a subcutaneous injection. He was given an initial course to last about two months.

Within a week the patient told me that mentally he was better than he remembers for 10 years. He continues to get positive feedback from family and friends as far as his mental status and speech. After a month all his body aches were gone. He was doing pull-ups with the biceps with no problem. The knee was pain free. The vertigo was not completely relieved but it was improved. An interesting aspect is that his acid reflux was gone.

The patient had an initial SPEC scan of the head in October 2019 which showed extremely poor cerebral circulation and decreased function in multiple portions of the brain. One month after the described treatment a repeat SPEC scan showed marked improvement in cerebral function and circulation. In fact, several radiologists at the imaging center had never seen such rapid improvement in any patient. And this correlates very much with the patient's subjective reports.

I adjust the dose of the BPC 157 depending on the patient's presentation during the healing process. A longer course of the BPC 157 could be used, or another peptide instituted down the line. Other patients given the BPC 157 have also reported improvement in gastrointestinal symptoms, and the acid peptic complaints disappeared with this patient. I will continue the BPC 157 for two more months.

Peptides can be a part of the wound healing process themselves or combined with stem cell therapy. My practice is not one that patients come in to get a shot of stem cells and receive a bill. I monitor the patient many times through one or two years as we go through rehabilitation and direct their treatment based on the personal healing response. Peptides can be an active part of this. Biohacking.

Basically, the philosophy is rebooting the cells to work normally. Peptides play a part. In addition, so is the use of biologically active NAD, exosomes, and stem cells.

Regeneration leads to rejuvenation. Cells function more optimally. Rebooting cells is more than just an oil change. This is an overhaul. Personal maintenance is so important.

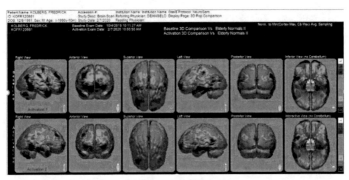

This image is pretreatment. Blue indicates no profusion, green minimal and yellow optimal blood flow. The red on cerebellum shows optimal output.

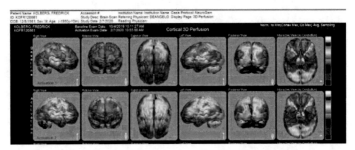

This image is post treatment. It shows significant improvement in blood flow and brain function.

When the body's cells are restored to work more normally, the body functions better. This isn't accepted in conventional medicine, but in my practice I will reassess and continue on with a further game plan for the patient.

The main thing to notice in the above graphics is that the 2nd shows an increase of brighter colors which equals more brain activity. The treatments and procedures applied to this particular Navy SEAL rebooted his physical body and increased his mental acuity. This represents an improvement of the whole human machine.

And it is important to keep these experienced 55-year-old military guys going strong. They allow us to all sleep in bed at night.

The other common peptide that is used in my rejuvenation program is epitalon. I have one patient who eight years ago had a baseline chronological age of 62 and a biologic age of 56 using telomere measurement. Following a health program and a year after a course of epitalon with a chronologic age of 70 the patient's biologic age was 54 using the same telomere measurement. Biologically younger. That is me below.

Reboot. Regenerate.

https://www.linkedin.com/pulse/can-you-get-younger-joseph-edward-bosiljevac-jr-md-phd-facs/?trackingId=YpvD-sqqJ80moEutzbWJdzg%3D%3D

https://www.linkedin.com/pulse/benefit-rejuvenation-joseph-edward-bosiljevac-jr-md-phd-facs-1f/?trackingId=Y7x9O8C DIJEd0Uuemqg%3D%3D

https://www.linkedin.com/pulse/beat-coronavirus-joseph-edward-bosiljevac-jr-md-phd-facs/?trackingId=77JI%2FoEd-Czqco%2B1%2Fw%2Fl%2Fkw%3D%3D

https://www.linkedin.com/pulse/peptidesa-summary-joseph-edward-bosiljevac-jr-md-phd-facs-1f/

https://medicine.wustl.edu/news/surprising-culprit-nerve-cell-damage-identified/

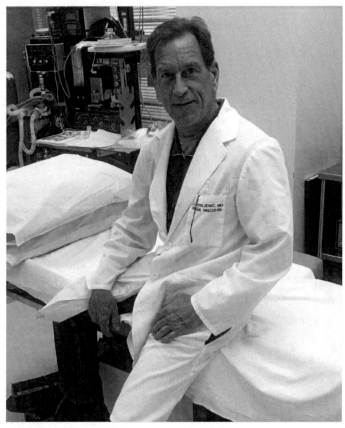

Dr. Joe's goal is to reboot the lifestyles of individuals so they can live longer, more active lives.

26

I Pondered Weak and Weary By Corbin Bosiljevac

It finally happened, all at once. While it should have been expected, I was not prepared for the adventure of a lifetime that I was about to embark upon. I could never fully be ready for it, but here it was staring me in the face.

Federal Prison was my fate.

Looking back, I learned more in those 7 years than I ever could have imagined. This was a vacation that I never wanted but was not going to be allowed to miss for anything. To deal with your innermost fears on a daily basis with nobody to help and no break to gasp for air should wear a person out. But God never gives you more than you can handle if you simply trust.

In prison I experienced the personal growth that I yearned for through college and corporate America. It took adjustments, but the end result is a product of mental stability that I couldn't get through years of strife in the workforce.

The quote, "Fear is the mind killer," as stated clearly in the 1980's sci-fi movie 'Dune' is a reality in every facet of life.

This is no joke. It paralyzes. It reminds you of how others perceive you and then scoffs while you slump in your own shame. Fear hinders whatever task you attempt, but only until you accept it.

More than anything it is a device of destruction that causes inaction while missing out on the present, the only thing that is important. Seeing that movie as a kid, this quote stuck with me as I have fallen victim to fear throughout my life.

Until I experienced the most frightening thing to me, something that I never expected to do, I didn't understand how to live in this world. I only existed in it but did not LIVE in it. There was a place that not only frightened me; it caused anxiety attacks when faced with its real possibility of becoming my future.

When I was finally led behind locked doors by Federal Marshalls, my world became heavy and fear collapsed my skull. 5 minutes were hours and every nervous twitch and movement was magnified since I was the new guy. Every worldly item was taken from me and I was no longer able to identify myself by things obtained in life. It was only my character, my poise, and my trust in God that would define me from this point on.

It took a long time in there, years really, to understand my fear of life and to appreciate our place in this world without anxiety. When I finally began to envelope myself into my worry is when I began to finally live. I was 38 years old.

To delve into these topics in more depth read my book, "On to the Next Thing." This chronicles my growth through accounts and anecdotes. It isn't just about the changes; it's about the stories along the way that truly bring humanity to those who struggle.

Fear, it is powerful and paralyzing. It can be a motivator or a handicap. While making you strive, it invariably tears you down and we are none the wiser.

What I'm saying here is that fear, along with truths and uncertainty, are the dominating factors in determining where our lives will lead.

So, the best way to deal with fear is to live in it. Just like we must live in the world, not near it or around it, but IN IT. We can rely on temporary measures to carry us through, but it is our presence that makes our lives real.

I apply this to our current world condition where people are scared because of the coronavirus pandemic. This situation has shaken the country to its core, and it is not only about sickness. It's about jobs, economy, grocery stores, social gatherings, holidays, and our way of life. We are all experiencing first world problems that are weighing a load on all of us.

Suddenly everything has changed, and the uncertainty has left us all in a different space of understanding. Some are concerned about wearing masks while others revel in mask ridicule.

Some are still quarantining while others want to go out into the world and live free as Americans have known for centuries.

Many Americans are still giving virtual high fives while others are back to hugging with social distance already the least of their concerns.

Masks, gloves, quarantine, and social distance are all measures that eventually lead to fear. These are temporary solutions for living in the world. Permanent solutions are what we are aiming towards when we refer to 'Survival on an Island.'

It took time away from society for me to appreciate it and overcome my worry for the world. Now I can view the societal changes of 2020 as simply adjustments to life as we know it.

The part that I am taking more seriously is what is under my control, and that is my <u>health</u>. Specifically, I am focusing on my immune system, cellular makeup, hormone balance, and functionality of my human machine going forward. If I do the best I can to keep my biology running optimally, then the constant shifts in the world around me are easier to accept. This certainly keeps my fears subsided realizing that health always comes before money.

CB

Dr. Joe's view on fears: This kid taught me so much about serenity. Mine is now better because of Cory. Fear? My brother Tim and my son Cory have lots of experience—I try to learn, but it is hard to listen to my 'little brother.'

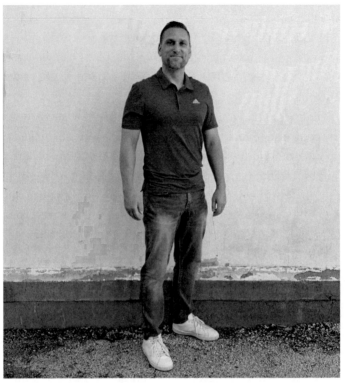

Corbin Bosiljevac at age 44. Living in the world means healthily confronting your fears.

27

The Start of the New Normal

9 May 2020

1. Stay-at-home orders are relieved in some places, but not here in New York City. May 15 is the reevaluation day.
2. The Empire State building had blue-and-white lights supporting the New York Police Department in their effort with coronavirus.
3. As the weather warms the viral load should decrease. California, Texas, Georgia, and Florida are easing some restrictions in this first step of recovery. We can see what happens. In New York City the weather has been cool and damp—corona environment.
4. I am looking for a new office and sometimes wonder if I will be able to make it to the end of the year with practice expenses piling up. I have not seen any SBA money.
5. Pedestrian activity is increasing, and everyone wears a mask.

6. Street traffic may be up to 35-40 % of normal during workweek. Weekends are 25%.

7. I've been doing antibody testing on patients here in Manhattan. Half the patients that are positive with corona antibodies never had any symptoms or illness. 1% of patients overall here in Manhattan have positive corona antibodies.

8. In some areas clients are waiting up to two or three hours in line to enter a Home Depot.

9. My girlfriend had the time to go through the change jar and made $243.18. She told me none of the coins had my initials on them—how could I make a claim? The ravages of coronavirus!

10. Hospitals are having less corona patients admitted and are able to manage the load. With better control the Javits hospital closed and the USN Comfort sailed home to Norfolk. The death rate in NYC continues at over 200 a day this past week. Some elective surgeries will be permitted in hospitals now but not in private office operating rooms.

11. Long-term projection is not easily predicted. This is a new virus. Novel medical treatment is used and results reviewed. The individual as well as society in general need to be considered. We are playing a ballgame—not quite halftime.

12. Will there be a relapse?

It is important to follow hygiene precautions. Almost every individual needs to reboot the system to be more healthy. If you are obese, have high blood pressure, diabetes, and heart or lung conditions the chance is less likely to survive a coronavirus infection.

More things to consider:

- The first part of the "Survival on an Island" book series is e-published this week.
- My son, Corbin is working on this with me. He has presented some aspects as far as anxiety. His history is one that dealt with fear—he is a survivor.
- I opened up my eyes this AM. Ha! Life could not be better.

Here is something that gave me perspective as we are not quite 2 months at this point into the pandemic measures taken by the government. Foreign ships coming into the New York harbor 200 years ago were required to quarantine for 40 days with all sailors remaining on ship to be sure that no illness arose. How did they pick 40 days? Well, this covers the incubation period for most infectious diseases. Also, after 40 days there was no way the sailors would stay on board! Think about this in terms of the quarantine with the local pandemic. After 40 days patience wears thin. Is this time period similar to what happened again here in 2020? Are we moving forward simply because we are becoming restless or because we understand what to do now? 40 days…

https://www.theatlantic.com/health/archive/2020/04/pandemic-confusing-uncertainty/610819/

https://www.bbc.com/future/article/20200421-will-we-ever-be-immune-to-covid-19

https://www.linkedin.com/pulse/coronavirus-testing-can-come-back-i-get-again-what-me-joseph-edward/?published=t

28

Local Epicenter Report: Manhattan, NY

15 May 2020

When I moved to New York City 12 years ago I felt that it was reasonably clean. Today, the subways are closed from 1 until 5 AM for cleaning and disinfection. Homeless are not allowed to sleep on the train. I was in the subway a week ago and there was a Hispanic man with no mask spitting out on the deck surface. In this area New York City has improved cleanliness. Traffic in the subway is down. The deal is how the city will pay for all of this.

Central Park is about ~30% normal capacity. Some of this may be the lack of tourists or visitors. Today it reached 82° accompanied with an occasional soft cooling breeze. It is sunny with protective ultraviolet rays. This is my hiking at the present times since I will not go camping this year. I like looking at the plants and I saw a cherry tree with baby cherries the size of a tiny pea.

Later I am sitting on the balcony of my apartment. I live

about a block away from the subway and this is about 4PM on a Friday. Pedestrian and vehicular traffic is about 30-35%. More than half of the vehicular traffic are service vehicles. Very little personal use of automobiles is noted. By 8 PM Friday night things are quiet.

The office is not open. Occasionally I see a single patient using isolation precautions. I have been doing antibody serum testing in the office. I make a home visit once or twice a week. There are a lot of phone calls and emails. Occasionally I will use Skype, but I just don't want to have someone see me sitting around in my pajamas.

Everyone is wearing a mask. This may not be done correctly but this encourages people to improve personal hygiene. There is minimal talking and conversation with masks. People appear to be less friendly. The bellman is always surprised when I come by and give him a big good morning. Grocery stores control crowds. On the sidewalk there are small stop signs 6 feet apart for people in line. One person comes out and one goes in. Inside shops cash counters have plastic windshields for protection and 2-foot white boxes placed near the counter to keep you farther away. However, they still touch your money using rubber gloves that touch a lot of money. One of the frequent measures of the spread of microorganisms is money. Another is a cell phone. I have seen people wearing a mask and gloves, playing with a cell phone, and then adjusting the mask with their hand.

I have been doing antibody testing in Manhattan. Positive antibodies are seen in 1% of local inhabitants. Of the 1%, one half of the patients tell me they have not been sick for years. Other family members in each household where there were patients with positive antibodies never were sick and none had positive antibodies.

29

Truths, Fears, and Uncertainty

20 May 2020

- We are still not at halftime of the corona pandemic.
- Will there be a second wave? Or over by November 11?
- Uncertainty with this epidemic leads to anxiety.
- Honest and valid information, misinformation, and disinformation are all available.
- Disinformation leads to anxiety.
- Economic consequences for New York City residents are very significant.
- To deal with anxiety, take certain steps and reassess.
- There continue to be advances in antibody testing.
- Improvement of personal and social hygiene and overall health will improve resistance to virus infections. This is key.
- Some complaints in this country may be called first world worries.

Dylan Murphy, an infectious disease modeler at Princeton, tells us that the long-term is like modeling the trajectory of a falling leaf, but the short-term is like a falling bowling ball. We still are not at halftime of the Corona ballgame.

This fall, particularly October or November, there may be a second wave.

And there is a rare case where a woman from Texas was infected with virus a second time.

This has not been the only coronavirus in our history which was also seen with SARS and MERS (cousins to the current virus). There are over 500 different coronaviruses. Most of these are found in bats and recent studies have indicated that perhaps 10,000 more different coronavirus are present in bats. For virus survival there are a lot of mutations. This is a zoonotic virus. In other words, it can transmit between people and animals. The contagiousness of this virus is not completely understood. The formation of antibodies is also a key.

Saskatoon, Saskatchewan demonstrated that bats carry the virus with no illness and the wet markets increase the risk of human spread. In my opinion, Louisville slugger *Carl Yastrzemski* bats are the best.

It will be impossible to prevent all further virus epidemics. SARS and MERS are examples of epidemics that were controlled. Viruses are part of the normal world. We cannot wipe out all viruses. Viruses will never be eliminated. It is necessary to live with the virus long-term. We need to adapt and survive.

As my son Corbin said, we must live IN the world and confront our current life with a more permanent solution. Antidotes and vaccines are solutions, yes. But those are things that are out of our control. Your personal health IS under your control.

Were we wrong about how we dealt with this back in March? No. Just no experience, particularly with the contagiousness of this particular virus. This is causing social anxiety. There are unknowns regarding the new pandemic. Pandemics demand depth and breadth of expertise. Our country has not been through anything like this in our lifetime, although the Hong Kong flu in 1968 was bad.

A vaccine is not yet available although advances are being made.

Social media and the Internet carry a lot of information. Scrutiny is needed because many assume that anything out there is fact. Many papers are being published but not scrutinized for validity. The information presented should help with clinical management and recovery. Misinformation and disinformation. Fake news. Increased anxiety.

Understand that I'm not trying to tell you what to believe, but I am saying to take action into those things that are under your control. Your health being one of those.

An example of reliable information is the balanced and unbiased manner in the article written by Ed Yong for the Atlantic magazine.

Not all literature available is valid. He points out a comment where Mr. Bergstrom indicates that pandemics fall in slow motion. In today's society many people want an immediate answer, treatment, and no mistakes. There are still some unknowns. Scientists at Singapore University of Technology and Design estimate the coronavirus pandemic in the US will end by November 11.

CAMBRIDGE, England — *The United Kingdom is among the hardest hit nations regarding COVID-19 infections and deaths. Now, a new study out of Cambridge University suggests that not enough is being done in U.K. hospitals to identify hospital staff infected with the coronavirus.*

Researchers tested 1,200 supposedly fit-for-duty National Health Service staff members at Addenbrooke's Hospital last month, and 3% ended up testing positive for COVID-19.

All patients admitted to British hospitals are immediately screened for the coronavirus. However, NHS staff, including patient-facing workers like doctors and nurses, are only tested for COVID-19 if they display relevant symptoms. We all know by now that individuals can be contagious carriers of the virus without exhibiting obvious or even subtle symptoms.

Among the 3% who tested positive, roughly 20% didn't feel any symptoms at all, 40% admitted to very mild symptoms that they had shrugged off, and another 40% said they had felt some passing symptoms over a week ago that had gone away.

I have short-term experience performing serum antibody testing here in Manhattan using a finger stick blood draw and a test strip where an answer is available in 10 minutes. 1-2% of patients in Manhattan test positive for the Corona antibody. One half of these people have had no recognition of any illness or symptoms. What does this help us decide?

If antibodies are positive, then the patient is at no risk for spreading the infection or being infected. If there are no antibodies, then it is important to use a mask and personal hygiene which helps protect others. It is important to improve personal health to increase resistance. Getting past this coronavirus is not to say another type of virus would come on down the line.

Numbers at this point indicate that 95% of patients develop antibodies within 2 weeks of illness.

This is a new virus and encourages learning a lot of epidemic and immunologic treatment with this current illness. Other work on monoclonal antibodies and a vaccination is in the works, with a good portion of this being done in Europe. How about llamas providing an antibody that may be helpful?

An effective monoclonal antibody may have been developed in Israel. For this reason it is important to stay up with the international literature as far as world wide thinking outside the box. Summer weather may decrease the viral load but there is concern about a second wave in October or November.

The virus may change little around the world, but the presentation can vary a lot. There are genetic differences and climate variance that play a part.

ICELAND

Case study notes:

Iceland's chief epidemiologist, Thorolfur Gudnason, said the approach's success is shown by the fact that about 60% of people who tested positive were already in quarantine after being contacted by the tracing team.

Kari Stefansson, deCODE's ebullient CEO, said the approach showed that "with the use of modern science, even an epidemic like this one can be contained."

Iceland's testing yielded new leads for scientists about how the virus behaves. Early results suggested 0.6 percent of the population were "silent carriers" of the disease with no symptoms or only a mild cough and runny nose.

Some calming and logical advice proposed going forward can be this: Take social as well as personal steps that appear to be appropriate at this time. Then provide reassessment at intervals. This may help us learn how to play the ballgame from here. Learn as you go and remember to live in a functional world going forward. Not a world that lives on pause or in sputtering starts and stops.

To overcome this coronavirus does not guarantee another there may not be another epidemic in the future. This is where personal health is key.

PERSONAL HYGIENE

Start with improved personal hygiene. Washing hands is the most important. There is more risk with exposure indoors so masks should be used in a closed space. Bathrooms are one of the biggest risks. There is a lot of discussion whether surface contamination is significant. We continue to learn.

How about clothes and shoes? Taking shoes off at the door is just a good overall practice here in New York City, particularly after walking out on the busy sidewalk with people and a lot of dogs. I never practiced this in the Midwest. I would drive my car into the garage, close the door, and routinely walk into the house. I really had not spent a whole lot of time with my shoes on an outside sidewalk. When my girlfriend tells me to take my clothes off and shower, I do not argue.

Subways are also part of this closed space, but New York

City has really picked up the maintenance and disinfection. Subways are closed 1-5 AM for cleaning. They are as clean as a plate coming from a dishwasher.

Improved measures of disinfection with regards to opening stores are addressed later in this article.

Personal maintenance is needed to reset the human machine to improve resistance and recovery. The goal is to get cells functioning better. Other treatments may include biologic agents that can be rebooted in all cells after they have become depleted. Reboot your cells.

PERSONAL HEALTH

A big step toward resistance is improving personal health. 60% of Americans have a significant health problem. Obesity, diabetes, smoking, high blood pressure, and stomach problems may be more or less controlled with medications. That does not mean that the person is healthy. These processes lead to things such as heart and lung problems, kidney trouble, a faulty immune system, and a detriment for complete healing.

One third of all fatalities were in nursing homes.

Viruses are part of this world. Did this catch us off guard? How much of this pandemic attacks patients who are not resistant or have a difficult time recovering from an infection? Personal hygiene with a whole food diet, routine disinfection and other measures are integral. After this virus is handled there is no guarantee long term for protection from another virus. Personal health and personal maintenance are key. Treat your human machine like a car.

The Betadine or iodine PVP-1 nose spray is an effective

disinfectant developed by the British. This is a simple and inexpensive antiviral measure. Coronavirus attaches to the lining of the throat. Iodine kills viruses. President Trump referred to Clorox for disinfection. What <u>he really meant</u> was iodine. Chlorine and iodine come from the same chemical family, but iodine is a healthy heavy metal. It kills viruses that tend to line the nose, mouth, and throat. A dilute solution can be used to spray nostrils and the mouth. The effect lasts for about three hours. This can be used after someone has been out in public for a while or exposed to some undue exposure. The healthcare workers in England used this on a regular basis when on duty.

GLUTATHIONE

Case presentations are helpful and I remember morbidity and mortality conferences regularly held during my surgical training. Learn from experience. This case presentation shows thinking outside the box of conventional medicine. It introduces the concept of using glutathione.

Glutathione is important. Any antioxidant supplement will work through several steps but at the tail end of any cycle of oxidation it forms glutathione which is the cells' master antioxidant. As far as an antioxidant supplement, start with glutathione itself. This is fairly straightforward. Glutathione plays a vital role in many metabolic functions.

There are chronic conditions where low glutathione levels serve a significant factor. These include cancer, Crohn's disease, ulcerative colitis, resistance to chronic diseases such as HIV/AIDS. Muscle fatigue and skeletal muscle wasting our symptoms of depleted levels.

Glutathione promotes cellular health. It inhibits viruses. The antiviral quality is that rebooting cells leads to improved cell function including the immune system. It can affect the natural killer cell activity so it boosts the immune system.

Remember I am a biohacker. I like to use biologic substances to restore normal metabolic activity to cells. When cells function normally the result will be increased health and resistance. This is rebooting cells.

I have used up to 1000 milligrams of glutathione intravenously on patients at any one time. When cells function normally there is improved health and resistance. After age 50 we all need an overhaul. An oil change is not enough. Getting older can be so subtle, but it still can be slowed or reversed.

Coronavirus can cause serious lung problems. The case summary tells about a medical student who took the advice of Dr. David Horowitz, a Lyme disease specialist. He recommended 2000 mg. Glutathione leads to break down of mucus so it is not clumped together. I will not get into scientific details about glutathione— there is other literature out there. It cannot be absorbed well by mouth, and fortunately worked in this particular case. IV infusion is best, although liposomal glutathione would also be effective. A source I trust is **Quicksilver Scientific**. A clear liposomal solution contains smaller liposomes that are absorbed better. Sublingual is convenient and can be very effective. My final comment - Dr. Horowitz, what a brilliant judgment call demonstrating your experience and ability to think outside the box.

VITAMIN D3

Another aspect is the use of vitamin D. Experiencing sunlight with ultraviolet rays can eradicate viruses. In addition, this may improve vitamin D levels, which also has an antiviral effect. Ten minutes is a good exposure.

There continues to be more data coming out regarding the importance of vitamin D with immunity.

Some common preservatives such as sodium benzoate can interfere with the conversion of vitamin D2 to D3. We are not receiving enough vitamin D in our processed diet. Even a whole food diet may be deficient depending on the environment in which it was raised.

I have patients in Florida who continue with low vitamin D levels despite sun exposure. The most important aspect is the goal expected from treatment with vitamin D. It should improve bone density, sugar metabolism, and has a tremendous anti-inflammatory effect. The effect depends on the dosage. There is no flat dose or level for everyone. Look at the goal of the treatment.

The current reference ranges of vitamin D may not be optimal. Or perhaps the physician accepts a vitamin D level at the lower end of the conventional range as being acceptable when a higher level would be more beneficial. Many patients do not usually have any or repeat testing for vitamin D blood levels.

Because a vitamin D level is within the normal range it may be accepted. Patients requiring ventilator assistance for lung problems with corona many times have low vitamin D. So do black patients who are notoriously prone to low vitamin D levels have higher morbidity?

My presumption is that only 50% of Americans have optimal vitamin D3 levels-what is best for them. *Vitamin D is in the hormone family!* This is significant! This is discussed further when we look at hormone optimization.

VITAMIN C

New York hospitals are treating coronavirus patients with high doses of VITAMIN C. Dr. Andrew Weber says he has been immediately giving his intensive-care patients 1,500 milligrams of intravenous vitamin C. The Long Island-based pulmonologist and critical-care specialist with Northwell Health says patients are given three to four doses a day.

The regimen is based on experimental but promising treatments that were done in China.

Jason Molinet, a spokesman for Northwell, says Vitamin C is being 'widely used' as a coronavirus treatment throughout the health system.

A clinical trial into the effectiveness of intravenous vitamin C patients with coronavirus was conducted on February 14 at Zhongnan Hospital in Wuhan, China.

Vitamin C is frequently in the news as far as fighting colds, flu and infections. The preferred method is whole foods. There are molecules in an orange similar to but not exactly vitamin C. The synergy of the various substances in the whole food makes this a preferred choice as the best way to take vitamin C. Only so much vitamin C can be taken by mouth before it is excreted by the kidneys. For infection and to decrease inflammation would require intravenous administration of about 20,000 mg. You cannot take that much vitamin C by mouth.

Another very effective vitamin C formulation uses liposomes as a delivery agent. **Quicksilver Scientific** is a good company for liposomal products. There is nothing special related to the coronavirus as far as vitamin C. However, it can help counteract the inflammatory effect in our body as a result of the infection.

IV clinics are available for vitamin C where 20,000 mg is infused over a period of a couple of hours. In the New York case 1500 mg was being used every 6 hours. Liposomal vitamin C is well absorbed and leads to good intracellular vitamin C levels for 12 hours from a 1000 mg sublingual dose.

MONOLAURIN

Coconut oil contains lauric acid. This is converted by the human body into monolaurin. Monolaurin as a supplement taken in a daily maintenance dose of 3000 mg has a potent antiviral effect. This can be increased to three or four times a day if symptoms occur. Another alternative is to take a couple tablespoons of coconut oil as a maintenance dose and increase that to 3 or 4 times a day if symptoms occur to help overcome an infection. This can be purchased online and a good source is *healthnatura.com.*

TRACE MINERALS

Let us look at another area of personal health that is not covered much with conventional medicine.

Case Study notes:

*The study's principal investigator **Ahmad Sedaghat**, MD, asso-*

ciate professor and researcher for the University of Cincinnati's College of Medicine, said in a statement that 61 percent of COVID-19 patients surveyed reported "reduced or lost sense of smell." *Comparing this to their other reported symptoms, researchers were able to draw some possible conclusions.*

"If the anosmia, also known as loss of smell, is worse, the patients reported worse shortness of breath and more severe fever and cough," Sedaghat also said.

Loss of smell may also help doctors determine how long a patient has been infected with the virus, which is useful information for determining treatment.

"If someone has a decreased sense of smell with COVID-19, we know they are within the first week of the disease course and there is still another week or two to expect," Sedaghat added.

Many coronavirus patients have the symptom of loss of taste and smell. With my surgical background I learned when patients reported this postoperatively that it was due to zinc deficiency. The symptoms respond many times within a week with additional zinc supplementation. My point here is that mild trace mineral deficiency, particularly zinc, may allow more susceptibility to viral infections. These are subtle things about our health that may be significant. It is nothing that makes us go to the emergency room for anything urgent. But this many times represents what society accepts as 'you are just getting older.'

Trace minerals are not routinely measured in conventional medicine. There is a device called the **Oligo scan** which gives results within minutes examining tissue levels of various minerals as well as toxic heavy metals. This is a good way to obtain a baseline evaluation and can be used in follow-up to consistently follow tissue levels due to supplements or other therapy.

A good example would be iodine. This is important for thyroid function. Sometimes patients may have suboptimal thyroid function in a manner that one day the thyroid works a little bit better than other days. Optimal thyroid activity can come and go during the course when the patient is slowly losing thyroid function because of some disease or condition. This can fool the doctor if blood work was drawn on a given day where the thyroid is working better. It does not confirm that the overall thyroid function is suboptimal for that patient. I have seen thyroid blood levels fluctuate in patients who are not stable.

I have also seen patients who have been on thyroid medication and begin to have hypothyroid type symptoms. Listening to the patient is the key. Are there symptoms suggestive of low thyroid? I check iodine levels. If this is low, then supplementation alone may restore proper thyroid function. Over 75% of patients I tested have low levels. If iodine levels on these patients are low, my first recommendation is to take 2500 μg a day. This is well above what is "recommended." Accepted ranges accepted in conventional medicine may not be optimal.

An excellent source of iodine is liquid sea kelp iodine. Remember this is a healthy heavy metal. If thyroid cells are deficient in iodine, then the thyroid may not function well daily despite prescription medication. Iodine repletion improves thyroid function. With this step I have seen patients come off the thyroid medication a couple of years after initiating a program to replace depleted iron stores.

Depleted cells can have these minerals restored as a part of a rebooting program. Low zinc is a subtle sign that may lower immune function. A zinc and copper ratio show how minerals coordinate together. Copper is important with many enzymes and is very supportive of heart muscle health. It helps protect the immune system. It also keeps hair from getting gray.

There is also a level between copper, zinc, and magnesium as far as ratios for optimal function. Some heavy metals such as selenium and iodine are very good for our health.

A whole food diet with appropriate nutrients and trace minerals is at least 80% of our health. It is important to keep cells healthy. Reboot cells by restoring healthy biochemicals to the cells so they function optimally. Adequate hydration and optimal trace mineral supplementation needs to be considered as building blocks.

Biohacking is the new buzzword of 2020. If you can take control of something in your life, then your health is of great importance going forward. By taking control of yourself with small incremental changes to what you eat, your quality of sleep, what you put into your body (food, liquid, supplements), how you move (exercise, stretching, posture) then you are becoming the best you possible.

Biohacking for me is rebooting cells to work better. Glutathione, vitamin D, trace minerals, and iodine all can be used to balance the entire "human machine." Conventional medicine does not have the time or experience, but these things can be a very subtle aspect of your health that affects aging and resistance. These are key to rebooting cells, personal maintenance, and rejuvenation.

Mineral balance is one of the simple but essential keys to personal health. This is frequently ignored in conventional medicine and current medical literature.

There are a lot of trials with hydroxychloroquine and Ramdev sivir I am no expert, but I do not believe there are magic bullets right now. Also, some of these magic bullets that you see marketed heavily may not work well if the personal health is suboptimal. This is the overall key.

Testing can determine if the body is healthy and free of viruses and more optimal for cell rebooting. Serum antibody testing in the office using whole blood from a finger stick test can give an answer in 10 minutes whether the antibody is present or not.

If the antibody is present, there is no danger of recurrent infection or spreading. The question comes up about the danger of reinfection in the fall even if antibodies are present. I do not see this is any major issue. Advances in vaccinations are being made.

How long do the antibodies last? In medical history these have been protective and according to the usual routine of viral illness and should continue to protect for at least a few years and provide herd immunity. Will this help if the same virus or a mutation comes out in the fall? The antibody testing may be false negative early so after 3 to 4 weeks following an infection would be the appropriate time to test for serum antibodies.

If no serum antibodies are present, I propose a protocol for patients based on personal hygiene. This will be coming and can include repeat testing in the fall as needed.

BUSINESSES OPEN-SOCIAL HEALTH

Right now, the epicenter for the current pandemic is still New York City. There will be regional variations as far as incidence and resistance. The most important aspect is social distancing as businesses open. So, limited clients are the plan. With a small personal business continued hygiene is important.

Clorox is an effective disinfectant— but can be toxic to us. Try to keep as organic as possible. Consider the following as an effective multi-purpose cleaner:

- Thymol essential oil - 20 drops. This is an effective antimicrobial as good as Clorox.
- 2 cups purified water, 1/2 cup citric acid powder. Use this on heavy use surfaces as this won't weaken your personal immune system.
- Also, a little vinegar spray on clothes and furniture can be used to sanitize and make things smell fresher.

CONSCIOUSLY MOVING FORWARD

The next step in recovery is adding travel, locally, regionally and including international travel. Many small businesses with restricted space, the bathroom, or an airplane promote an environment more likely for contagion. Subways are also part of this closed space, but New York City has really picked up the maintenance and disinfection. Subways are closed 1-5 AM for cleaning. They are as clean as a plate coming from a dishwasher. More ultraviolet lights will be seen in public facilities.

Herd immunity for COVID-19 may not be so far off after all, this new model shows.

Religious facilities reopen with restrictions.

An aspect where I hold no expertise is the economic

recovery in New York City. Hotels, restaurants, movie theaters, and entertainment activities are completely stopped. Restaurants can deliver or provide take out. This is a big economic depression. It took 10 years to get past World War II and about 10 years to bounce back from 9/11. This is World War III with corona. This is not an overnight issue. Economic pressures can cause mental stress which leads to physical symptoms that may not have been experienced before. It is extremely important to now view the whole human machine (mind, body, and soul) as part of a wellness stability program going forward.

If handled appropriately from the contagious standpoint and if a vaccine becomes available quickly, we may be able to cut down our economic bounce back to under 10 years.

HOW ABOUT THEM DAWGS!

Another significant aspect that could positively affect how we can operate large, crowded events would be the use of dogs. To help monitor areas both before, during, and after an event they can use their sense of smell. Residual viral presence can be identified to help improve overall disinfection. Cleansing and disinfection is important. Ultraviolet lights will become more frequent. An effective way to provide better disinfection of a public place like the subway with a lot of volume may be with dogs. Perhaps the dogs can help prevent further epidemics.

I propose this as an important issue as we move ahead to open up large facilities and events. More ultraviolet lights will be seen in public facilities, but dogs can also be useful and key to getting us back to successful, safe public gatherings.

LAST FEARS

Homeschooling kids in the Fall? This is being proposed, particularly for the New York City area and can certainly add to anxiety.

NOT A SECOND BABY BOOM

FLORENCE, ITALY — *It turns out a global pandemic and recession isn't much of an aphrodisiac or incentive to* start a family. *Many have speculated that couples being stuck at home all day will lead to an influx of new births over the coming year, but a new study has largely disproven that notion.*

Researchers from the University of Florence conducted 1,482 online interviews on parenthood desires and beliefs during this pandemic, and over 81% of respondents said they are not looking to conceive *while COVID-19 is wreaking havoc across the globe.*

Moreover, 268 of the survey's participants admitted that before COVID-19 emerged on the world stage they had been planning on having a new child. Now, though, 37.3% of that group have shelved that idea for the time being. As far as why so many people have decided to put off starting a family, 58% are worried about the future economy and another 58% expressed concern about possible coronavirus-related pregnancy complications.

The survey, which consisted of 944 Italian women and 538 Italian men, was carried out during the southern European nation's third week of lockdown. All respondents were between the ages of 18 and 46.

Why the decreased libido? Stress may be related to the

middle class with limited savings and lost jobs. There are people that continue with salaries but working from home and having the house full of kids can be frustrating. The decreased libido appears to be in general. No one is interested. What is happening is social anxiety. How does it affect each individual? How are relationships within the family? What is the fear of the severity of the disease? Beyond that there may be fears that I realistically would address as first world fears. In today's society many people want an immediate answer, treatment, and no mistakes.

What I see in mid-May is more social isolation. There are no friendly hellos behind the mask and many times people are looking at the ground. To say good morning is almost an intrusion on their privacy. I'm trying to take a little extra effort to just say good morning to people and also to stop and visit with the bellman. I do not shake hands.

New York has a reputation of being an isolated city as far as natives being strangers and isolated. After living here for 12 years I do not believe that is so. I feel people here in Manhattan are very friendly. However, the friendly activity between all of us that live here in the epicenter is not what was three months ago.

Also, look at the attitude from going back to a highly tourist district. As far as my New York City patients, half of them are living away in Florida are California. They may not come back for a while.

I passed a young woman who was pushing a stroller and walking with a child. A bottle rolled out from the stroller and I reached ahead to pick this up for her. She actually shouted, "do not touch that bottle!" as it rolled into the street. This demonstrates some of the social response that has developed. Less personal. She assumed that me touching that bottle would be more detrimental to her health than rolling around in a New York City gutter.

I see people are less sensible and personable. Much of this sensibility refers to disinformation. I'm trying to provide good coaching, but the patient is the one who plays the game.

In today's society many people want an immediate answer, treatment, and no mistakes.

That is where I hope we can grow as a society to overcome these fears.

There are still some unknowns.

How about opening gyms?

This is the 20th of May.

https://www.dailymail.co.uk/news/article-8330301/112-coronavirus-cases-linked-fitness-class-South-Korea-asymptomatic-instructors.html

https://www.prevention.com/health/a32368635/coronavirus-second-wave/

https://canoe.com/news/world/i-was-floored-texas-woman-gets-covid-19-for-a-second-time

https://www.dailymail.co.uk/health/article-8289011/Mutant-strain-coronavirus-make-infectious-dominant.html

https://www.studyfinds.org/super-immunity-may-explain-how-bats-carry-coronavirus-without-getting-sick/

https://www.bbc.com/future/article/20200421-will-we-ever-be-immune-to-covid-19

https://www.sciencemag.org/news/2020/05/unveiling-warp-speed-white-house-s-america-first-push-coronavirus-vaccine

https://www.theatlantic.com/health/archive/2020/04/pandemic-confusing-uncertainty/610819/

https://www.dailymail.co.uk/news/article-8350935/US-coronavirus-pandemic-early-November-predictive-model-shows.html

https://www.studyfinds.org/cambridge-study-3-of-hospital-staff-may-be-unknowingly-carrying-covid-19/

https://www.jpost.com/health-science/iibr-completes-development-phase-of-covid-19-vaccine-626913

https://apnews.com/b13115dba10ad0aa4f9e1f22a3403c

https://www.linkedin.com/pulse/16-april-i-came-across-release-from-british-group-joseph-edward/

https://drsircus.com/general/glutathione-against-the-coronavirus/

https://medicalxpress.com/news/2020-05-vitamin-d-role-covid-mortality.html

https://scitechdaily.com/vitamin-d-determines-severity-in-covid-19-researchers-urge-government-to-change-advice/

https://www.msn.com/en-us/health/medical/the-one-
symptom-that-predicts-how-bad-your-coronavirus-case-
will-be/ar-BB13QeKi?li=BBnb7Kz

https://www.sciencedaily.com/releases/2020/06/200624172050.htm

https://www.cnn.com/2020/05/22/politics/cdc-guidance-
religious-worship/index.html

https://www.studyfinds.org/not-now-study-disproves-
theory-that-coronavirus-lockdown-will-lead-to-baby-
boom/

30

The Girl from Honduras

I have made a total of 10 medical missions over the years. Being fluent in Spanish I prefer Latin countries. Each trip was for a one to two-week duration and I traveled to Honduras, the Dominican Republic, Colombia, Bolivia, and Mexico. Journals were kept and so I share a few memories here pertinent to the subject of survival in our world today.

It was necessary for me to bring a full set of surgical instruments on my trips and initially these were transported as my carry-on for the airplane. My trade tools were borrowed from the hospital operating room. Packing space was a premium. I tried to think of the most useful instruments and would also bring medications since these were always in short supply. With increased security concerns on later trips (after 9/11) the surgical equipment was handled with the general luggage. That always made me wonder if I could do my work once we arrived if the instruments did not. And then to have to face the operating room supervisor about lost instruments— well, we are talking in the range of about $50,000 or more (1990s).

Traveling by bus we arrive in an area, usually a rural part of the country, and set up. Sometimes this is an existing medical facility or perhaps an empty building. Local lay help is part of the team as well as medical personnel such as nurses. Our group also has its own lay help and paramedical personnel including a pharmacist. Sometimes there is a dentist. Other physicians from various specialties make up the remainder of the team.

On some trips we are also accompanied by military Special Forces that ride the bus and stay with us. Big guns are part of the cargo, but it shows the desperation felt in some areas. In a way it makes you feel like a celebrity. The local people are excited for the arrival of foreigners from far away. Instead of giving out candy or money, I gather children around me. I carry a book consisting of photos of my family, home, and countryside where I live. It includes a map so they can see from where we come with relation to their country. I have even been invited to come in and talk to the children in their schools.

The first full day is spent setting up the clinic. We will not begin operating for three or four days yet and the OR takes longer to be prepared. Members of our group were skilled in electrical, plumbing, or carpentry and building improvement. They did plumbing, ran wiring and some construction so that after we leave an empty building can be used as the clinic going forward and provide a local medical facility to the community. Our presence there is meant to be a perpetual boost for them and not simply a one-time medical event.

So, the military guys will not teach me how to shoot their guns. Well, I will not show them any surgery!

I feel pretty comfortable since I speak Spanish well. I help with directions and communication between our crew and the local community. My deficiencies won't be noted until later.

So patients are seen the first two or three days in the clinic and scheduled for surgery. There is exposure to diseases and conditions that are not seen in our country except in textbooks or perhaps going back to that one year spent at Charity Hospital in New Orleans for my medical internship. Some patients need additional preparation or outside exams prior to surgery. They are offered necessities such as dressing material and simple medications like Tylenol or Pepto-Bismol. I try to explain things in lay Spanish terminology and some patients really stretched my knowledge of Spanish slang. I would like to share with you four of my best experiences.

This 23-year-old male comes in with an inguinal (groin) hernia. For me, an inguinal hernia is not a big operation. This patient tells me he is not employable with the hernia. He has a wife and two children. He traveled by bus for five hours to see me. His surgery was done using local only anesthesia and the next morning he was out the door on the 9 o'clock bus for the five-hour trip to go home. He took a packet of 2 Tylenol in case he might need it during his bumpy ride.

This experience changed his life in that by removing this ailment he now has the opportunity to seek out work, thus providing better for his family and increasing their happiness in the world.

Next, a 34-year-old gal needed her gallbladder out. Obviously, on a mission like this we do not have the capacity to do laparoscopic or minimally invasive surgery. So, I made an incision below the right rib cage and performed an open gallbladder operation.

My daughter Kristin was with me on this trip. She had just started college and looking at going to Veterinary school. After I made the incision, I told her to put her hand on top of mine and slide her hand inside the abdomen. Then I guided her so that she could feel the anatomy including the stones in the gallbladder. That is quite an experience to have your oldest daughter be the first assistant in surgery! An interesting note is that Kristin finished medical school, a residency in family practice, and a one-year fellowship in sports medicine. She finished a final fellowship in mommy hood and has a three-year-old daughter.

The next day I went to the female ward to make rounds before starting my day. I looked around and saw my patient standing in the corner helping someone make their bed. Patients would bring blankets and sheets from home. Food was provided by families and much of this was fresh produce, and the local staples of rice and plantains. I noted the same in the large metropolitan hospitals.

Anyway, I walked up to her and asked if she was hungry. She said yes. I asked her if she was having any pain. Her answer— "Well, of course, I have pain - I just had surgery yesterday." She probably went home to do the laundry for the family after I dismissed her the next day. I think she took a total of two Tylenol the first 24 hours and only because it was offered. Something as simple as Tylenol was not affordable for many of these patients.

Thinking further about gallbladder surgery on these missions, my youngest patient for this procedure was 11 years old. That is another story.

Now, I speak Spanish pretty well, right? I can talk with the local people and relate with my Latin colleagues on a professional level. So, this 13-year-old girl is brought into the clinic by her grandmother. She has a hard lump the size of a medium orange in the lower third of her thigh. I felt this and knew immediately it was a bone tumor and was worried it was malignant. They were given a slip of paper to get an x-ray.

They returned two days later and after looking at the x-ray I saw that this was a benign tumor comparable to a mushroom growing on a narrow stalk off the main bone. I am not a bone cutter, but I am a good surgeon. This could be trimmed off, so to speak. I was smiling when I pointed to the bump on her thigh and told her and her grandmother, we would take her to surgery and get rid of this. I was speaking about the benign tumor. I tried to keep it simple and on their level. In Spanish.

We did not have all the instruments needed. Looking around, one of the members of our group showed me his carpenter tools. Before the case, a small hammer and a chisel were cleaned and sterilized which allowed me to complete the procedure successfully. The carpenter and I were both beaming!

Later that day on post op rounds I found her crying and asked what was wrong. She said to me "Is it gone?" I nodded and said yes, playing the role as a confident American doctor. Through the blanket I touched the bulky dressing placed in the operating room after surgery. She began to cry again and said something about losing her leg. I asked her to lift up the blanket and when she saw both feet she smiled and wiggled her toes. This little girl and her grandmother thought I was going to amputate her leg. In a roundabout way I had finally made her day.

The final episode is one of my favorites. A pretty 18-year-old girl comes into the clinic. When she was two years old, she had the hair and scalp covering the entire top part of her head ripped out after her hair was caught in farm machinery. She had a bald area the size of a medium pancake. Surgeons and pathologists frequently compare things to food— whatever that means. So, what I intend is a circle of bald scalp about 6 inches in diameter.

Anyway, looking at her I said "Sorry, but I cannot do anything." She turned to leave the clinic and began to cry. The "big" American doctor could or would not do anything for her.

One of the local Honduran nurses there had worked with me on previous trips. She came and punched me on the arm and said "Doctor, do you know what you just did? This little girl is considered damaged goods and will never get married. Can't you do something for her?" So, I walked outside the clinic and found her crying with the waiting crowd. We went back in and I began to play around with her scalp.

There is a layer of connective tissue that attaches the scalp to the skull. This allows the scalp to move around a bit. If this is divided the skin can actually be advanced one or 2 inches and has the capacity to stretch a bit more after that. I told her I could not close the entire deficit, but the gap could be reduced to maybe one and a half inches. Yes, yes, yes, yes, yes!!! She beamed with hope.

So, we go to the operating room where music was set up to make her comfortable. The procedure will be done entirely under local anesthesia. What I used would last 6 to 8 hours. Most of these patients require very low doses of any medication.

I did a circumferential injection all the way around the base of the scalp at ear level. After that I could start dividing the connections between the scalp and the bone and begin to slide the skin up over the top of the head. Starting at each end I put in a stitch that would dissolve after about a month. We would talk, laugh, and tell stories while waiting a little bit to allow the skin to stretch some. The entire procedure took about two hours. She was left with a silver dollar size deficit. Today, she wears her hair long and nobody knows. Three children now trail after this Girl from Honduras. And the procedure will delay the development of forehead wrinkles. She will look young longer.

These people are so grateful and compliant. Pain management is not known as a specialty here. To minimize swelling I asked the Girl from Honduras to sleep with her head up on three firm pillows for 10 days. I know these instructions will be followed to the letter.

As I said before, none of what I did was lifesaving, but much of what I did was life changing. We had to improvise. Sometimes MacGyver would have been proud. I learned that I can operate with my head, heart, and then a knife, fork, and spoon. So, what if you lose the surgical instruments - except having to face the operating room supervisor!

Was it worth it? I lost that time in office income and still had my overhead expenses. I paid my own way for the trip. Such was a small price to pay for another adventure in my life. No question it was worth it. What a bargain!

31

Personal Prevention

OBSERVATIONS ON MAY 23, 2020

- Religious facilities reopen with restrictions.
- Although public drinking is strictly prohibited, there are people on the sidewalk with masks off drinking in front of a restaurant with delivery.
- Once a day early evening there is a parade of bicycles several blocks long on 2nd Avenue and also playing loud music like a concert.
- FDR Drive Thursday evening was very crowded. This was right before the weekend holiday with people traveling.
- Many want to go to the beach. New Jersey beaches are requesting that New York people stay away. The New York beaches are not open except in Nassau County.
- For the first time in 2 months I see some airplanes and even see an occasional helicopter.
- Sitting on the balcony I watched from above a father teaching his son about safety as the child rode a skate-

board. Good father!!

New York is starting to increase commercial activity. Anxiety grows when there are unknowns. However, healthy positive steps can be taken on an individual approach. Here are some simple preventive measures to consider as far as personal health:

1. Personal hygiene is a responsibility, particularly handwashing and touching mouth, nose, or eyes. The virus attaches to the lining of these areas.
2. Masks and gloves should be used appropriately depending on exposure.
3. Betadine or iodine PVP-1 nose spray. This is a simple and inexpensive antiviral measure. Coronavirus attaches to the lining of the throat. Iodine kills viruses. A dilute solution can be used to spray nostrils and the mouth. The effects last for about three hours. This can be used after you have been out in public for undue exposure.
4. Hong Kong and Japan are recovering without shutting businesses and a total lockdown.
5. Herd immunity is obtained by everyone encountering the virus followed by recovery and antibody formation. Antibody testing including repeat antibody testing down the line may be useful in understanding contagiousness, distribution, and resistance in society and give information on treatment approaches in this pandemic. Universal testing may be available for us to see and understand this epidemic better. What is learned can be protective for future viral pandemics.

6. Vaccinations or maybe a monoclonal antibody effective against coronavirus may be available this fall.

7. Ramdev sivir may be an antiviral treatment that can be helpful in severe cases. There are no magic bullets.

8. What is frequently neglected when things go well are personal health measures of <u>rebooting and rejuvenation.</u>

9. Reboot cells to function more optimally. Cells wear out with time. Get an overhaul not just an oil change.

10. The reason why there is so much media coverage about youth and immunity is because there is a connection, in general, with a younger body and the strength to fight off sicknesses. This is true with many ailments, not simply coronavirus. A younger body is fresh and vibrant, able to take on the toxicity of the world. Over time, body parts wear out, including the immune system and the organs that support the human machine. What I am proposing here is to get younger, to stretch out the usefulness of our human body in order to have a better well-being and enjoyment of life.

11. Scientists at Singapore University of Technology and Design estimate the coronavirus pandemic in the US will end by November 11.

12. Continuing is the second part of my list of preventative measures to consider going forward in our uncertain world:

Dexamethasone has shown it is helpful (end June). This is a tremendous anti-inflammatory agent. The lung problems that occur are due to an increased inflammation reaction. The dexamethasone can settle this down so the patient does not develop swelling that impedes absorbing oxygen while breathing.

There is concern about a rebound epidemic in the fall. There is no guarantee another viral epidemic will not occur in the future even beyond the present. The key is personal health for prevention and recovery. Will we play offense or defense?

We are almost at halftime for the coronavirus game. It is time to reassess and decide what steps to take right now in the ballgame.

Increased personal health promotes resistance and recovery. Here are some simple measures that are quite helpful in recapturing your health.

Coconut oil contains lauric acid. This is converted by the human body into monolaurin. Monolaurin taken in a daily maintenance dose of 3000 mg has a potent antiviral effect. This can be increased to three or four times a day if symptoms occur. You can always do a couple tablespoons of coconut oil as a maintenance dose and increase that if symptoms occur to help overcome an infection. This can be purchased online. A good source is *healthnatura.com*.

Receiving sunlight with ultraviolet rays can eradicate viruses. In addition, this may improve vitamin D levels, which also has an antiviral effect. Ten minutes is a good exposure. We have seen the current coronavirus as still prevalent in the summer months although the outdoors can be safe when social distancing is in play. It is the close proximity that leads to clusters and breakouts.

The effect of vitamin D has been very important and emphasized during this pandemic. History and experience in my profession has shown me that blacks are notoriously low in vitamin D3 levels. Location, background, race, and social life are all things I consider when doing a blood work panel and compiling my plan for each individual's healthy lifestyle plan.

https://www.linkedin.com/pulse/blacks-corona-joseph-edward-bosiljevac-jr-md-phd-facs/?trackingId=K6grwc%2BzTLuKUI

https://www.linkedin.com/pulse/monolaurin-viral-infections-joseph-edward-bosiljevac-jr-md-phd-facs/?trackingId=RJGh%2BI-hZJVmJh3tJKHKDew%3D%3D

https://medicalxpress.com/news/2020-05-vitamin-d-role-covid-mortality.html

https://www.linkedin.com/pulse/unique-aspects-vitamin-d-joseph-edward-bosiljevac-jr-md-phd-facs/?trackingId=7%2Fggq0M hvGrdwGTofB9VA%3D%3D

https://www.studyfinds.org/study-how-hong-kong-managed-to-contain-covid-19-epidemic-without-total-lockdown/

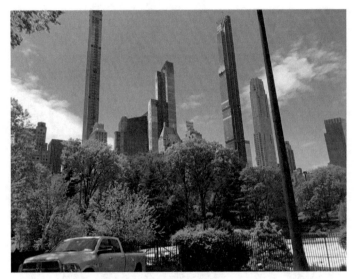

May 15, will the city be able to keep it's real estate occupied?

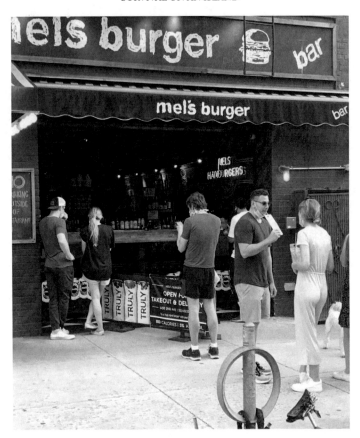

Friday night take out.

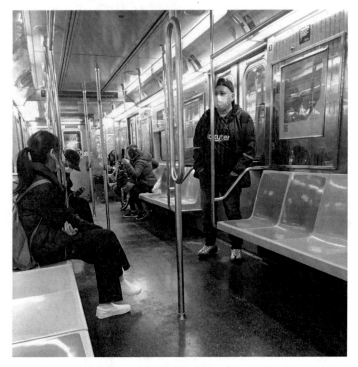

Subway crowd, mid day May 4th.

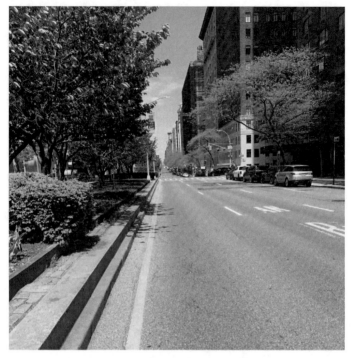

Park Avenue at 2pm on May 15.

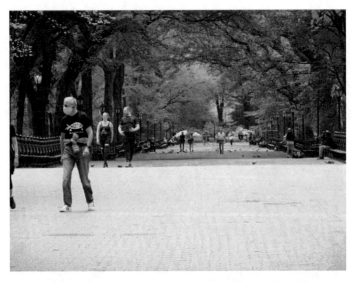

Social distancing in Central Park on May 15.

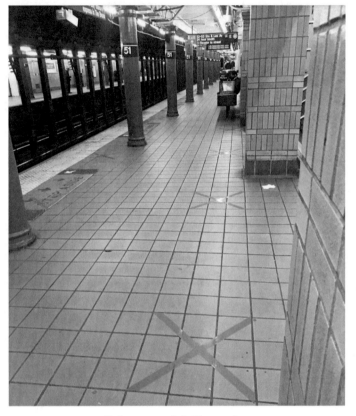

Subway social distancing.

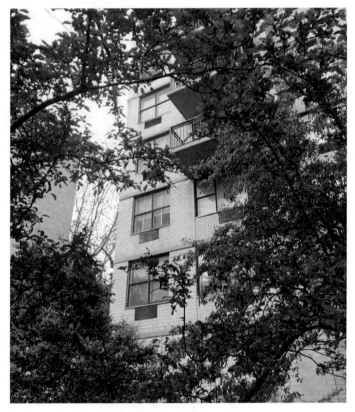

My 4th floor balcony refuge.

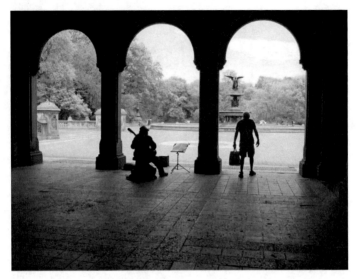

Central Park musicians.

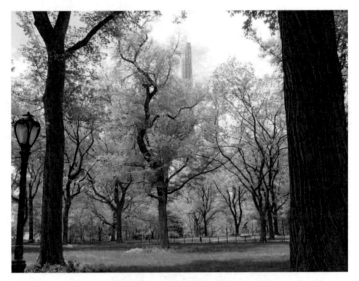

A beautiful spring day on May 15th in the park. The natural world worries not about our pandemic.

32

Using Antibodies from Llamas to Fight Coronavirus

I have mentioned previously that wartime and major illnesses have contributed much for our medical knowledge.

The function of the immune system is intricate and the possibility to control more aspects can help not only with infection but also cancer.

200 years ago, when ships would approach a harbor, they would sit off dock for about 40 days. This is the way quarantine was handled in those days before entry into this country. This appeared to manage the lifestyle of infectious diseases. It was also about the maximum amount of time that you can keep sailors on deck when they were in port.

At the time this is written we are about 40 days out from the social isolation in NYC. There are a lot of protests as far as easing social restrictions, the opening of beaches, retail shops, and restaurants. This is very similar to the time length as far as the sailors waiting to ship in quarantine. Is this just one of the human characteristics? This pandemic is teaching us a lot not only about medicine but also lifestyle and society.

40 days is about the patience threshold for humans and this hasn't changed in generations.

One of the big goals in defeating the coronavirus is to establish a vaccine to produce an antibody that will neutralize the virus. Vaccinations for SARS CoV1 and MERS CoV have not been developed in humans. Waiting for a vaccine may take time and therefore it is important to have Plan B and Plan C...and moreover implement these plans so you can live in the world.

A group out of Austin, TX working with Belgium has taken two copies of special antibodies found in llamas and used these to create a new antibody that neutralizes the coronavirus, or COVID-19, in humans.

"This is one of the first antibodies known to neutralize SARS-CoV-2," says co-senior study author Jason McLellan, associate professor of molecular biosciences at UT Austin, in a release.

"Vaccines have to be given a month or two before infection to provide protection," McLellan explains. "With antibody therapies, you're directly giving somebody the protective antibodies and so, immediately after treatment, they should be protected. The antibodies could also be used to treat somebody who is already sick to lessen the severity of the disease."

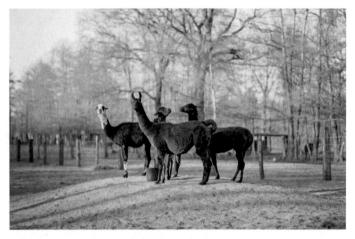

The immune system of llamas could teach us a few things.

https://www.theguardian.com/world/2020/may/03/happy-hypoxia-unusual-coronavirus-effect-baffles-doctors

https://www.studyfinds.org/an-unlikely-ally-llama-antibodies-key-to-potential-covid-19-treatment-breakthrough/

33

On the Brink of Summer

28 May 2020

1. Alternate side parking was suspended until June 7. People have been allowed to park on the street without charge for the past 2 1/2 months. In that period of time a person may have saved $1500 in parking garage fees.
2. My hair is getting longer, and I look like Joel Osteen. There is a lot of diversity in New York and so I don't appear a lot different than many despite my nose. Barber shops are still closed.
3. There is evidence that the BCG vaccine for tuberculosis may be protective with the coronavirus. The benefit is to improve the general immune response.
4. I am sitting on the balcony almost every night and note in all the other buildings there was no one else sitting on the balcony. And I mean every night. I have had a balcony with my apartment for many years. Less than 5% of apartments have balconies. Once in seven years have I seen another person sitting on a balcony. The

weather is warm, and I enjoy making phone calls and doing paperwork outside. That is the closest to outdoor camping I will get this year unless I go over to Central Park to wander.

5. The Giants and Jets facilities have opened in New Jersey with restricted staff. I went over to see Joe Namath and was told "Just leave, old man."

6. Streets are 70% full. Restaurants are not open. Almost everyone is wearing a mask.

7. Just keeping up a little sociability I try to talk with the bellman. Those masks tend to have people acting more private and secluded. Not even looking up or a good morning. Once, worrying about getting my mask ready, I forgot to zip up my pants.

8. Union Square and Times Square have been empty. For the last couple of days what started with peaceful demonstrations after the death of the gentleman in Minneapolis last night was accompanied by looting and destruction of property.

9. Public drinking is strictly prohibited. Ha! Ha!

10. June 1st Gov. Cuomo and Mayor Bill de Blasio placed an 11 PM curfew over New York City. Philadelphia did the same starting at 6 PM. Washington DC is 7 PM. We are the older adolescents.

11. Maybe smokable CBD could decrease the violence with the current riots.

12. The local Sprint and Verizon stores, which are located eight blocks away from my apartment, had all windows broken and were vandalized.

34

CBD and Corona

Much of the information coming out about this Corona pandemic is making people from scientists and doctors to businessmen and factory workers look at their place in the world a little differently. We are considering how to keep ourselves fit and prime for living going forward.

An interesting aspect of this novel virus concerns the receptor sites on cells called ACE 2. A high concentration of these are found in the throat and lungs, the white part of the eye, and the testicles. ACE 2 receptors are more numerous in younger patients, decrease as we get older, and can be blocked by medication.

There are high blood pressure medications that work at this receptor site.

Some of the ACE 2 receptor activity is modulated by sex hormones so estrogen and testosterone may play a part. This is the gateway for coronavirus. It attaches at that site for entry into and infection of the body. That detail makes the ACE 2 receptor a hot topic right now.

This raises questions:

1. Does the number of these receptor sites influence infection with corona?
2. Is a patient that is taking medication blocking these receptor sites more at risk for developing infection?
3. How does CBD play a part?

I have pointed out that smokers have a lower incidence of Corona infection. When I first noted an outbreak of coronavirus in Milan as well as Spain I felt that this may be due to the fact that there is a higher population of smokers in these countries. Then I read the attached article that demonstrates that cigarette smokers are one fourth as likely to develop coronavirus. Again, another medical twist that 2020 is throwing at us.

This is interesting since the most severe complications of coronavirus are related to the lungs. Could nicotine be doing this? Or is this just the toxic smoke killing the virus? Just an observation as I attempt to learn more from this current pandemic.

So, my thinking expands to CBD. ACE 2 receptors can be modulated by CBD producing an anti-inflammatory effect. Can this help block the gateway for entry of the coronavirus? Is this another productive use for CBD?

What does this mean? This is not a magic cure to defeat coronavirus by smoking pot. But, this simply demonstrates the mechanism of biologic activity, particularly things that influence the ACE 2 receptor. Many of the medications that affect these receptors are administered for high blood pressure and heart and blood vessel problems. These may affect receptor sites and could influence the infection rate but this has not been noted to be a major problem. Patients are directed to continue their medications and not change these during the pandemic.

Smokable CBD did not change the violence in NYC last night.

https://www.dailymail.co.uk/health/article-8246939/French-researchers-plan-nicotine-patches-coronavirus-patients-frontline-workers.html

https://www.ibtimes.com/coronavirus-treatment-cannabis-enzymes-could-help-block-gateway-covid-19-study-2979422

https://www.statnews.com/2020/04/10/coronavirus-ace-2-receptor/

35

Early June—Recovery Begins

A patient of mine lives in Florida on the West Coast near Naples. There they have not closed down beaches, restaurants, or bars. As medical offices opened, she went to the dentist. They followed a certain routine checking temperature and asking specific questions as per protocol. She encountered a face shield and other protective type equipment.

Following that she went to another medical office. She does not like to take elevators and the office was on the second floor. Instead, she took the stairs wearing a mask. The first thing (within 5 seconds) they did when she entered the office was to scan her forehead with an electronic thermometer. The temperature was above normal and that caused excitement. They told her she needed to get out of the office immediately. She explained that she had been living by herself the last two months with no visitors and she just took two flights of stairs That made no difference to them.

We will see more episodes like this as we get back to

recovery. Sometimes we are <u>damaged goods</u>. The emotion and level of concern differs from person to person. While the intuitive person will remain calm, be smart, and carry on there are others that fear everyone else's actions while forgetting to take care of their own business.

In the world we cannot control others, as much as some people would enjoy it. Again, we can control how we approach the world and care for ourselves safely. My son tells me that it feels good to continue to move forward enjoying life, because time doesn't stop. He is cautious and thorough while adhering to respectable rules and suggestions about all health standards around the country. He also values time because of the things he has survived in his life and so he still lives every day happy and free. I see that the fear of this pandemic has not conquered him as it has others. He tells me that health is what keeps his fears low.

1 June 2020

Demonstrations and rioting began Monday when a store lost a large number of Rolex watches.

I heard there were over 300 protesters arrested, one being the daughter of the New York mayor. He released all of them immediately.

Tuesday all of Macy's windows were boarded off.

Curfew was 11 o'clock on Monday and changed to 8 o'clock in the evening on Tuesday.

2 June 2020

Tuesday there were five police helicopters lined up facing

west above my apartment here on the upper East side about 5 PM. There was a crowd gathering at Central Park.

One of the local restaurants is boarded up.

The Sprint and Verizon stores on 86th Street (7 blocks away) were broken into. All windows were broken and we will all suffer a 5G backlash.

This is a matter of "just be careful." I do not need to go to Union Square, Times Square, or Central Park, particularly after 4 o'clock in the afternoon.

3 June 2020

There was quite a 7 PM concert of quarantined citizens tonight that was really better than any we've had for the past month or so. There were cymbals.

After 8 PM there was no traffic below 96th St. here in the Upper East Side. You can walk in the street except that it is after curfew hours. I am inside.

I hear sirens as I sit on the balcony.

4 June 2020

2 PM There was a crowd on the corner below my balcony for the George Floyd Memorial. It stopped traffic on 2nd Avenue. Peaceful.

Later I'm sitting on the balcony doing paperwork and making phone calls. At 8 PM police cars with sirens went through the streets to be sure all traffic was gone. Again, no traffic below 96th Street was permitted.

5 June 2020

Things are picking up. The traffic is about 80% of normal. Pedestrian traffic is about 50%. Taking a walk by the East River I crossed FDR drive. This is busier than I have seen it for 2 1/2 months. This is probably close to 80 or 90% normal traffic perhaps because everyone needs to be home for the curfew and/or it is the weekend. This really has increased significantly.

On the street I passed eight policemen. This was at about 5 PM. They were next to a truck with two men. The back of the truck contained bricks in a package size of about 3 ft.² on a pallet. These were to be placed near areas of demonstration covered by a construction disguise. Protesters find weapons and window breaking tools from these bricks that are being planted for the riot.

Many go back to work Monday, **June 8th**. Primarily the blue class workers.

The Metropolitan Ballet is closed until December 31 and then they plan to reopen with a big new season.

Alternate side parking on the city streets will begin after 2 ½ months.

I give my prayers and sympathy to the family of George Floyd. Why do the media push this as genocide? We should all try to help each other.

6 June 2020

There is not much air flight noted. I enjoy telling my story from the epicenter of the pandemic. As a physician my goal is to teach patients how to be better. Personal health.

Tonight I actually see someone else sitting on the balcony. Well, it was for 10 minutes anyway. My balcony is my wilderness site and helps me relax.

36

Medicine is Science and Common Sense

We have covered some aspects of personal health. In my career I have kept long emergency room hours, worked in hospitals, performed surgeries and ran private practices. Through that time, I always valued personal long term health rather than only fixing immediate problems. Sometimes we did complicated things to get us 'over the hump.'

Let me give an example of a simple measure I learned.

As a surgeon I would oversee patients in the intensive care unit on a ventilator and make rounds on them three or four times a day. These patients received a daily chest x-ray as part of the early-morning assessment. One thing I sometimes noticed was a collection of secretions in one portion of the lung. This may be aggravated if the patient is stationary in bed. The secretions accumulate in the backside which further inhibits oxygen transportation. When this was seen, a change of the position of the patient was performed to prevent secretions or pooling in one location. This would also help mobilize secretions to be aspirated.

This is an example of a simple technique to deal with a serious issue the patient was dealing with. Turn them over onto their tummy.

I came across this article and it brought back memories. Can some more simple tactics be re-employed to help treat COVID-19?

The good news is we have been studying ARDS for over 50 years and we have a number of effective evidenced-based therapies with which to treat it," says Dr. Hardin in a media release. "We applied these treatments—such as prone ventilation where patients are turned onto their stomachs—to patients in our study and they responded to them as we would expect patients with ARDS to respond."

There was a fairly low death rate among the 66 patients that were treated using this method — 16.7%. Furthermore, after a follow-up period of at least 30 days 75.8% of these patients had been discharged from the ICU. It seems like using an ARDS treatment strategy is a good way to treat COVID-19 patients that are critically ill.

This is not a new technique, but it is many times ignored, particularly when there is an overload on the medical system.

So take this one step further. Ozone treatments are used to improve oxygenation at the tissue level. I have experience with this in my practice. Patients come in with an oxygen saturation of 93%. We go through an ozone treatment and 45 minutes later the oxygen saturation of 97% with no other change in activity or other treatment during that time. Oxygen heals and increasing its level in the human body promotes healing.

There are many scientific and medical facts that are being learned despite or perhaps due to the stress of an epidemic here in NYC. It can also re-emphasize certain known treatments and maneuvers that are simple and quite effective.

https://www.studyfinds.org/study-most-extreme-covid-19-cases-can-be-treated-with-standard-techniques/

https://www.linkedin.com/pulse/ozone-oxygen-therapy-coronavirus-bosiljevac-jr-md-phd-facs/?trackingId=t5aT-LOXbNlkPTkBGAuXHKA%3D%3D

37

Corona Dreams

The recent coronavirus has not hit us like the Spanish Flu, but the anxiety with the current pandemic is still significant. I was talking with my sister recently and she told me about trouble sleeping and bad dreams the last two months. Was the anxiety of her situation getting to her and affecting her dreamlife?

Since then I have asked several of my patients and many confirm this occurrence of bad or odd dreams. This is more evidence that the side effects of this pandemic are not simply health and money related.

There is other information out there about the significance of Corona dreams. The current thought is that this represents anxiety of the unknown, and part of this may be from a change in a daily lifestyle.

We are still learning. Many people would like instant information, immediate assistance, and no mistakes.

Do I have any special techniques for sleeping? Try Vegas. Every day I try to scan some of the lay literature for items of interest. This article about the Vagus nerve, really caught my attention.

Vegas is a name everyone knows. I wanted to spark your interest, but I am really talking about **Vagus**. The Vagus nerve starts out as one of the cranial nerves meaning it comes out of the skull. When I was in medical school I had to learn this acronym:

On Old Olympus' Tiny Top A Finn And German Viewed Some Hops

This helped me to remember the names of the cranial nerves:

1. Olfactory (smell)
2. Optic or ophthalmic (sight)
3. Oculomotor (moves eyeball)
4. Trochlear (same)
5. Trigeminal (sensation to most of the face)
6. Abducens (moves eyeball)
7. Facial (injury during plastic surgery causes sagging of the face)
8. Auditory (hearing and balance)
9. Glossopharyngeal (swallowing)
10. Vagus (the one we are discussing)
11. Accessory (muscles of the neck and shoulder)
12. Hypoglossal (wags the tongue—well developed in some humans)

So, the Vagus nerve comes out of the skull and just keeps going and going and going. It passes down through the neck to the chest and finally disperses branches in the abdomen. It goes to every internal organ between the skull and the hips. How important is that?!

Although this is a cranial nerve, the vagus is involved with sending nerve branches to every internal organ and every part of the body through the autonomic nervous system.

A ganglion represents a crossroad of nerves. The sphenopalatine ganglion (SPG) located above the cheekbone is such a crossroad and branches from several of the cranial nerves go through here. An injection of local anesthetic into this ganglion can cause a reset of the sympathetic/parasympathetic balance in the entire body. It can be used to break the cycle of severe pain with migraines but can also affect chronic pain in areas remote from the SPG.

The Vagus has some sensory properties, motor (means it moves muscle) function, and a lot of what belongs to the autonomic nervous system. This is a portion of our anatomy that works below our conscious level. There are two parts of the autonomic nervous system—sympathetic (which is related to fight or flight) and parasympathetic (a calming system for the heart and lungs and the ability to keep underlying functions intact, such as digestion and kidney function.

I want to introduce the concept of structure. This begins with the feet on the floor to provide the foundation. The structure then continues with ankles, knees, and hips, which function as two flexible pillars. These should be even in length and move symmetrically so that the pelvis on top is level. Above this are back vertebrae stacked like blocks. They tend to be a little more rigid in the chest portion because of the ribs. Once you get to the cervical vertebrae (neck bones) there is not as much rigidity and so there is increased potential for injury because it supports the weight of the skull and brain. The craniocervical junction is where the neck bones meet the skull. This is a potential weak spot during high velocity trauma.

Now why am I mentioning this? Physiotherapy, deep massage, and chiropractic adjustments can correct misalignments in the vertebral column. This, in return, can affect function of the vagus nerve. Peripheral stimulation can track back to the main vagus with a resultant reflex on another organ—such as slowing of the heart rate. Many stretching and yoga maneuvers can stimulate the vagus nerve.

The reset button is one of the more common things in today's society. Slapping the monitor on the side only works so much if I have trouble with my computer. Many times when something is not right, I just restart the computer. The same thing goes for other electrical devices throughout the house. Most of the time the reset button is just what is needed.

This also led to the use of the SPG (sphenopalatine ganglion) block in stem cells for addressing chronic conditions of the autonomic nervous system dysfunction.

As far as the procedure, it is a straightforward injection above the cheekbone. It can be done as an office procedure. And yes, I've had this done myself. It is one of my sacrifices for patients. I was dealing with chronic neck pain from an old football injury. The injection was done with lidocaine which lasts about 20 minutes. After the injection, I had this feeling of calm similar to drinking a glass of wine. The neck pain was much better for two or three days after that. I still occasionally have acupuncture and adjustments to take care of the neck, but it is 95% better long term.

So that led to the possibility of using the SPG block for traumatic brain injury or blast injury in military subjects. With my background and experience in conventional as well as natural medicine, I try to apply things in an overall picture of health. Stem cells injected into that area can give long-standing results and actual repair and healing as well as relief of pain.

I had a patient with chronic low back pain, and he did not like to take narcotics. Surprisingly, pushing the reset button by doing an SPG block can play a part in pain located some distance from the head. It worked here. Remember, the vagus nerve sends branches everywhere.

I get excited about all these things because many are so simple yet can have a very significant effect on overall health. I like to step outside the box. At the age of 70, I finally feel I am pretty good at this stuff. Observation and listening are an important aspect in my approach with patients.

I would caution you about the analogy of an SPG injection to a reset button. What really happens in humans? I don't think that this is an instant process but may allow parts of your body to reset and work from a new starting point again. In the computer this takes microseconds—the conductivity of electromagnetic energy through our own body is like 268 miles/hour (which is about 400 meters per second).

With humans, other modalities may be necessary for optimum effect. Here comes good nutrition, supplements, measures to lower chronic inflammation, psychotherapy, medication, the "human machine" concept or any analogy to a computer system is obviously limited, but it sure gets us into the ballpark. Look at below and compare the human machine to the infrastructure of NYC which needs stem cells.

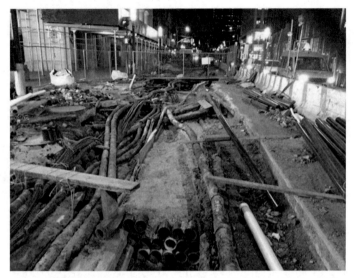

Wall Street and Broadway about 2015. Cover it up with concrete and nobody thinks about it. Needs stem cells.

So, if you are scared of needles, or want to consider another method that can be done on a regular basis to stimulate the SPG without going to the physician's office, here is an example:

There was a Dr. Milton Reder who practiced on Park Avenue 45 years ago. He was an expert at treating arthritis and other chronic pain by resetting the SPG. He did this by passing a long cotton-tipped applicator with numbing medicine through the nose to the back of the throat. He would position the swab and let it set for 30 minutes. His waiting room was full of people sitting there talking, reading, and every one of them with sticks up their nose. There still are a very few practitioners that can perform this technique.

His reputation was so good that many times a big politician, one of New York's most wealthy citizens, or a prominent physician would come in for treatment.

There was an orthopedic surgeon who tended to make fun of Dr. Reder. One day this doctor came to see Dr. Reder because of long-standing and persistent low back pain affecting his daily lifestyle. Dr. Reder was very good with him. As he positioned two swabs in each nostril, he muttered that it would be hard to keep two of those in place on each side. He tied a small helium balloon to each side. He then told the orthopedic surgeon to go sit in the waiting room at least 30 minutes. He was the only one with four swabs, two on each nostril attached to a balloon!

I looked at an ENT (ear, nose, and throat) textbook from the 1930s. SPG block by injection or with intranasal cotton swabs was taught to residents at that time. Then pain medications became common and this section is not included in modern texts. It is not taught routinely as part of an ENT program.

For home or daily treatment, mild pressure bilateral to the muscle overlying the "temple" over 1 to 2 minutes promotes further inhibition of the sympathetic nervous system of the Vagus. This promotes further relaxation and eases anxiety.

A very good exercise (that can be done along with the mild pressure) is to slowly breathe in through your nose as deep as possible, then hold this to a count of 10. Really take the deepest breath possible to the end of full inspiration. Let your breath out through your mouth slowly to that same count of 10. This maneuver stimulates the vagus nerve. It can improve anxiety, stomach upset, racing heart, bowel and bladder disorders and can even put you to sleep at night. I suggest doing this with three cycles of breathing 2 to 3 times during the day. One time can certainly be at night when your head hits the pillow. Ahhh! My pillow!!!!

https://www.webmd.com/lung/news/20200527/covid-and-sleep-sweet-dreams-arent-made-of-this?ecd=wnl_spr_052920.spr-052920_nsl-LeadModule_title&mb=lGVdiurmHB-MQOzQukn1aapAyWFWqf9PLEH%2foKnlpKv4%3d

https://www.thealternativedaily.com/vagus-nerve-health/

http://www.mhni.com/updates/sphenopalatine-ganglion-blocks-headache

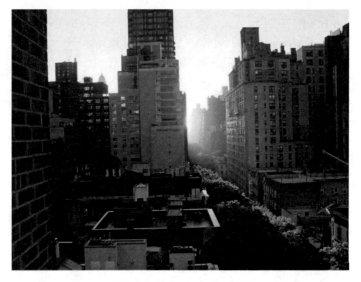

Manhattanhenge - July 13

38

Mechanisms of the COVID

There is a new silent symptom in COVID-19 patients and it's fatal.

Coronavirus is killing with SILENT hypoxia: Patients' oxygen levels fall dangerously low, but they don't have shortness of breath that usually signals the life-threatening condition.

Dr. Richard Levitan, an emergency medicine practitioner, said he saw COVID-19 patients with pneumonia come into the hospital with low oxygen levels. However, they weren't struggling to breathe, because they were still able to exhale carbon dioxide.

Physicians determined patients are suffering from hypoxia, which is when there are low oxygen levels in the tissues that can result in death.

Levitan recommends patients be monitored with a simple device called a pulse oximeter that measures oxygen levels before they dip too low.

This is a device that checks oxygen levels and could be an

early warning system for coronavirus as discussed in the article below. Any and all options should be considered. The latest is an adhesive film that makes a wristwatch a monitor. Interesting development.

Also, patients from high altitudes are likely to tolerate lung stress from corona.

Coronavirus can cause serious lung problems. The case summary tells about a medical student who took the advice of Dr. David Horowitz, a Lyme disease specialist. Glutathione leads to a breakdown of mucus so it is not clumped together. I will not get into scientific details about glutathione - there is other literature previously in the document. 2000 mg was recommended for this patient and she improved dramatically with this dosage.

In short, it cannot be well absorbed taken by mouth but this patient responded to the treatment. IV infusion is best, although liposomal glutathione would also be effective. I give 1000 mg per dose intravenously. A source I trust for the liposomal product is *Quicksilver Scientific*. A clear liposomal solution contains smaller liposomes that are absorbed better. Sublingual is convenient and can be very effective.

My final comment—Dr. Horowitz, what a brilliant judgment call demonstrating your experience and ability to think outside the box!

https://www.dailymail.co.uk/health/article-8245373/How-coronavirus-kills-silent-hypoxia-Patients-experiencing-life-threatening-oxygen-drops.html

https://www.studyfinds.org/ucla-scientists-develop-adhesive-film-to-turn-your-smartwatch-into-metabolism-monitor/

https://nypost.com/2020/05/09/new-york-mom-with-coronavirus-saved-by-medical-student-son/?utm_campaign=iphone_nyp&utm_source=mail_app

https://www.dailymail.co.uk/sciencetech/article-8391329/People-living-high-altitude-resistant-coronavirus-study-claims.html

39

Home Medical Monitoring

There is a current case study (**March 20, 2020**) which was based on low oxygen levels or hypoxia. This led me to recall a case study of my own.

I have a friend who is a 50-year-old black Dominican male. He is in good health with very low body fat. He eats a healthy whole food diet, takes supplements, and also uses alternative health methods such as red light and sauna. One of my observations was that it took vitamin D 50,000 units a day just to get him into the upper normal blood level. I have had only phone conversations with Robert. My last contact personally with him was late February after I got sick—with H flu, not corona.

He became ill with no fever or gastrointestinal symptoms. He had no cough and just did not feel well. His wife is a registered nurse and she provides IV therapies for my patients. She keeps complete vital sign records on patients which includes measuring oxygen saturation. She began checking her husband. The oxygen saturation monitoring on his finger said 85% which is quite low and is significant to me as a doctor. During the night it drifted down to 82%. At rest he was not short of breath and not having any respiratory symptoms or cough.

He saw a physician in a 24-hour urgent center. The doctor said there was nothing he could do for him and he should stay at home. That night his wife noted an oxygen saturation of 75%. Clinically, I am concerned at 85% but 75% is critical.

He presented to another urgent care where the doctor looked him over and said he did not appear to have anything serious going on. Oxygen saturation was taken, and it was 75%. Robert was sent immediately to the hospital where he later tested positive for coronavirus.

He was in the hospital for about a week on oxygen. CT scan of the chest was completely negative for any pneumonia or other abnormalities. Right now, he feels significantly run down. His hemoglobin dropped from 13 to 9 because of lysis and destruction of red cells from the viral infection. Liver blood tests are elevated but this also is due to the viral infection and will resolve in 6 to 8 weeks. Oxygen saturation last night (30 March) at home was 97%.

What occurred with Robert is medically noted as a cytokine reaction. He was very healthy and when this vicious virus hit he did not get violently sick. His underlying immune system fought and overcame it. However, the immune system kept going and overwhelmed him with a toxic hyper reaction. This is where a big cortisone dose (Decadron) could be used to lessen the inflammatory reaction.

Now get this one. He has had 3 antibody tests since March—I did one of them—all are negative. Give me an answer for that.

An oxygen saturation of 75% was life-threatening to this young patient.

What medical devices do you need at home?

When I was a boy, I remember the glass thermometer that had mercury inside. And yes, I played with the mercury when these broke. That was basically what we had as far as monitoring the patient. Things are now very different. Over the course of my professional career of 45 years other medical devices have become very common at home. An older doctor here in NYC told me that his father, who was a doctor, stuck a thermometer in his mouth. He was early teens and did not want anyone imposing on his life. He bit through it in defiance.

What medical devices do you need at home:

1. Finger stick or skin patch blood sugar.
2. Blood pressure monitor.
3. EKG finger pads for looking at an electrocardiogram or heart tracing.
4. The oxygen saturation monitor.
5. Electromagnetic pads for pain relief and recovery.
6. CPAP machines.
7. Oxygen administration equipment including an oxygen tank.
8. Although I do not think this is a medical device, my friend said to his wife he wanted to be cremated. Later that day she told him he was scheduled for Tuesday.

https://www.linkedin.com/pulse/corona-patient-how-difficult-diagnosis-bosiljevac-jr-md-phd-facs/?trackingId=d6xX%2Bu

PEbaFaUYwaAA%3D%3D

https://www.health.com/condition/infectious-diseases/coronavirus
storm

https://www.oregonlive.com/coronavirus/2020/03/the-
coronavirus-turns-deadly-when-it-leads-to-cytokine-
storm-identifying-this-immune-response-is-key-to-patients-
survival-report.html

40

Hormone Balance

I am involved in a medical practice of age management which basically involves chemical and hormone balance to help the human machine work better. Start with this: my father at my age had 50% higher testosterone levels than me and my grandfather had levels 50% higher than my father. Why? The environment, the atmosphere with toxins. Processed water. Plastics and chemicals that are in our environment, like Roundup. All of these can cause a premature drop in hormones and are very important affecting our health.

Overall, males of the same age group in the 1950s had testosterone levels 40% higher than the same age group today.

Men and women both use testosterone and estrogen. Females suffer frequently from estrogen dominance. Women need testosterone and usually a boost in progesterone. Men tend to lose testosterone and the estrogen: testosterone balance changes to where estrogen becomes dominant in males. Men also need progesterone.

Sex hormones promote recovery and regeneration. They decrease with age although I argue that there is a premature drop because of toxic influences in our environment. When I look at differences in testosterone in my family I notice premature aging.

Sex hormones, Vitamin D, and cholesterol are all composed of a steroid ring. Cholesterol is also used to make sex hormones and vitamin D. Vitamin D is a hormone but is frequently overlooked as part of overall hormone balance.

Hormone balance and optimization improve cell function. Sex hormones are used by the body for resistance, repair, and regeneration.

Last week (May 2020), doctors on Long Island in New York started treating COVID-19 patients with estrogen in an effort to increase their immune systems, and next week, physicians in Los Angeles will start treating male patients with another hormone that is predominantly found in women, progesterone, which has anti-inflammatory properties and can potentially prevent harmful overreactions of the immune system.

"There's a striking difference between the number of men and women in the intensive care unit, and men are clearly doing worse," said Dr. Sara Ghandehari, a pulmonologist and intensive care physician at Cedars-Sinai in Los Angeles who is the principal investigator for the progesterone study. She said 75 percent of the hospital's intensive care patients and those on ventilators are men.'

WHY START WITH PROGESTERONE?

Females generally have higher estrogen levels. Low progesterone levels lead to estrogen dominance. Hormone balance for estrogen dominance is many times approached with additional progesterone.

Progesterone has a key function as far as neurotransmitter recovery, the immune system, and to balance estrogen effects. So keep this in mind as we talk about the other sex hormones, testosterone and estrogen. Progesterone is significant.

Think about puberty. For men, during puberty testosterone levels are sky high. So are progesterone levels. In medical school I was taught to ignore the progesterone with men since this was a female hormone. Blood levels drop to the basement by age 30.

In my experience, many males have issues with decreased libido, benign prostate enlargement affecting the ability to urinate, prostate cancer which has spread to bones, progressive hair loss, and decreased cognition which may be improved with progesterone treatment.

In 1991 the Woman's Health Initiative (WHI) Study looked at hormone therapy in many women and demonstrated increased cardiovascular events as well as gynecologic and breast cancer with women using hormones.

My comment is that the hormones used in the study were non-bioidentical forms. This is the key. The reason I start with progesterone is to confront estrogen dominance which is frequent in our society. This may be the most important of the three sex hormones. Progesterone stimulates libido in both men and women.

SEX HORMONE BALANCE

Why are sex hormones important? They serve as a repair, rebuilding, and recovery agent. Testosterone can decrease body fat and improve body composition. The advantages for women are to maintain body composition, maintain or improve bone density, improve cardiovascular health, balance mood swings, and improve libido. The key is using bioidentical hormones and balancing ratios between all hormones. There is no magic bullet.

Sex hormones improve the response for better resistance to infection as well as recovery. This is pertinent not only with the coronavirus but in the future because other viruses may occur.

Cholesterol is a precursor for the formation of sex hormones and vitamin D. If these levels are suboptimal blood cholesterol goes up. This is all part of normal aging - correct? So middle-age men begin to take cholesterol medication and something for blood sugar. I see this as a typical pattern for Americans.

Instead of beginning a cholesterol medication consider this as a signal that the basic metabolism is out of order.

If hormones are OPTIMUM metabolic responses occur that lower cholesterol levels and improve blood sugar metabolism. Basic bio hacking to keep hormones at a good level.

A rising cholesterol level will go down when there are optimal levels of testosterone and vitamin D. Hemoglobin A1C will also go down since sugar metabolism is improved with testosterone. Many diabetics would benefit from testosterone therapy. And it is cheaper than many of the diabetic medications.

In 1991 the Woman's Health Initiative (WHI) Study looked

at hormone therapy in many women and demonstrated increased cardiovascular events as well as gynecologic and breast cancer using hormones.

An estrogen product from horse urine and synthetic progesterone were part of this study.

My comment is that the chemicals used in the study were non-bioidentical forms. This is a key. Biologic substances cannot be patented. A side branch of the estrogen molecule is changed and the product can now be sold as a patented product.

The conclusion of the WHI study is flawed and this study does not consider bioidentical substances as a key item. Bioidentical hormones should be used to supplement hormone levels to optimize metabolic effects as far as function of the body. This is an example of a "clinical study" which is accepted by conventional medicine and pushed on to the public even though there is significant lack of validity involved with this study.

This is where patients believe to optimize hormones levels is bad. If your thyroid is off, it is very acceptable to take a hormone for this. It is certainly different as far as the sex hormones. This is very shortsighted. I think a lot of people consider hormones not appropriate if they may be given by injection. The problem being is oral replacement for sex hormones is not the best way for administration. Topical creams, an injection for testosterone, or implanted pellets are the common methods used today.

What is an acceptable hormone level? Rather than low levels, the goal is in terms of optimal levels. For example, testosterone 250 pg/mL is in the "normal range" accepted by conventional medicine. At the age of 50 if levels are 250 my question is - what was the testosterone level at age 30? If the testosterone level was 1500 at age 30 then this is a significant decrease and a very suboptimal testosterone level. The optimal part refers to metabolic effects and how the body reacts. This is about 15% of an optimal level to function metabolically at age 50. With age, patients may not be quite as active metabolically as years earlier. It may be hard to lose weight and results from exercise are minimal. Cholesterol goes up as does blood sugar.

Elevation of blood cholesterol and type II diabetes are aggravated when sex hormones are not optimal. A rising cholesterol level will go down when there are optimal levels of testosterone and vitamin D. Hemoglobin A1C will also go down since testosterone improves sugar metabolism. These are the metabolic consequences.

*This is all part of normal aging - correct? No, **it doesn't have** to be.*

So, a middle-age man begins to take cholesterol medication and something for blood sugar. Today society says that these are a symptom or sign of "getting older." Aging is subtle and therefore it is important to look at function. If hormones are OPTIMUM, cholesterol meds may not be needed.

This is basic biohacking - keep hormones at an optimum level. Function at a younger metabolism. Extend active life by decades. When you were thirty you did not need a cholesterol pill. There are metabolic corrections with lowering of the blood cholesterol and improvement of sugar metabolism when hormone levels (including vitamin D) are optimized for each particular patient.

That is where I come in.

CORONAVIRUS AND HORMONES

Male coronavirus patients with low testosterone levels are MORE likely to die from COVID-19, German hospital finds:

- A German hospital assessed the hormone levels of 45 COVID-19 patients in ICU.
- Found that the vast majority of men admitted had low testosterone levels.
- Testosterone may be able to stop the body's immune system from going haywire.
- Low levels of the sex hormone are unable to regulate the body's immune response, leading to a 'cytokine storm' which can be fatal.

Sex hormones improve the response for better resistance to infection as well as recovery. Hormone optimization is important for wound healing and regeneration.

This is important not only with the coronavirus but in the future as other viruses arise since infection may be increased when men have a low testosterone level.

Men with low testosterone have increased risk of a severe cytokine storm, which is a type of exaggerated immune response producing significant inflammation which is harmful to the body itself.

Women appear to be more protected from a Corona infection, possibly on the basis of high estrogen levels.

A question that is not answered here —- what was the testosterone level in the females? Women with higher testosterone levels may resist and recover better from coronavirus? Or is it estrogen? Or a testosterone and estrogen ratio? I point out variabilities that may negate the significance of the results in some studies as well as to stimulate further thinking. An abnormal estrogen and testosterone ratio in men increases risk of prostate cancer.

ACE 2 RECEPTORS

Coronavirus CAN enter the body through the eyes: Scientists find eye cells are a prime target for the deadly virus to attach to:

- The coronavirus latches onto ACE-2 receptors, known as the 'gateway' into cells.
- Johns Hopkins University School of Medicine found ACE-2 in the eyes.
- It means if infected droplets land on the eye, the virus can begin infiltrating.
- This may also explain why some patients have suffered conjunctivitis.

Professor Nick James, of London's ICR, said: "One of the proteins the virus appears to bind to in lungs is TMPRSS2."

"It's a sort of lock and key thing: having bound to this protein, it provides the virus with a route into the cell."

Wide-scale use of the drugs as a coronavirus treatment "would almost certainly cause more harm than good", he said.

The Office for National Statistics (ONS) has recently released data which shows men had a 'significantly' higher rate of death from the virus than women in all of the older age groups.

Scientists also believe men may be more likely to die because their blood contains higher levels of an enzyme used by the virus to infect healthy cells.

Angiotensin-converting enzyme 2, or ACE 2, is found in organs like the heart and kidneys - and is thought to play a role in how COVID-19 progresses into the lungs.

Right now, I am presenting this ACE 2 receptor information pertaining to coronavirus, although these receptors have a widespread influence with our systems. This is part of identifying and understanding some of the metabolic pathways involved with good health.

Related to corona, ACE 2 receptors are found in good concentrations in body cells like the eye, the throat, lungs, as well as the testes. The incidence of these receptors is high in a young person which may improve their resistance to infection. Receptor numbers drop with age just like many other things. Women have more receptors than men.

It appears that sex hormones also work at this receptor site, which is where the coronavirus will attach. Although there is not a black-and-white answer, this may be one of the mechanisms that the body uses to protect itself from infection.

The coronavirus is always displayed as a round ball with spikes like a crown covering it. These spikes are the ones that attach to these ACE 2 receptors. It is their gateway to enter the body and produce infection. These are mechanisms that help understand the biologic pathway. Some of what is learned with Corona may not relate to current treatment, but learning more about the biologic pathway can improve overall medical knowledge.

Can blocking this receptor affect infection with coronavirus?

An important aspect is that hormone balance may interfere and block these receptor sites. As far as overall resistance, an improved immune response is also supported by sex hormones.

So, corona infection can be related to ACE 2 receptors in general as an entry site but no specific treatment related to the coronavirus has been shown. This was also shown with CBD which appears to affect ACE 2 receptors.

All of these facts lead back to the idea of keeping the human body hormonally balanced and physically and mentally fit while boosting the immune system. This isn't just to fight coronavirus, it's so a person can enjoy longevity of life with less fear or anxiety with any future environmental or societal issues.

Patients with severe cases of COVID-19 are often those with hypertension and either type I or type II diabetes. Many patients with congestive heart failure and hypertension take medication that binds to these receptor sites. Can the ACE 2 pathway alter risk for infection? This has been suggested but not answered with COVID-19.

There is no definite evidence that continuing to take medications which inhibit the ACE 2 receptor increases risk for corona infection. Certainly, the medications are being given for a chronic condition. My recommendation is to continue to take these medications on a regular basis. Do not change this because of the current epidemic.

I emphasize the fact that ACE receptors are seen in the eye to reinforce the fact that personal hygiene measures need to be continued, with emphasis of bringing a hand up to your eyes or mouth.

I did not understand the significance of the ACE 2 receptors in the testes, except increased expression can lead to kidney and testes problems including cancer.

Pulmonary-wise, blocking this receptor improves outcomes with ARDS (adult respiratory distress syndrome).

Other medications used for corona treatment may present a health risk. Hydroxychloroquine has shown cardiovascular effects perhaps tracing back to ACE receptors.

Ramdev Sivir has been associated with lower blood pressure and an irregular heartbeat in some patients possibly related to the ACE 2 receptors.

https://www.studyfinds.org/new-research-shows-how-coronavirus-can-take-a-dangerous-toll-on-the-heart/

https://dnyuz.com/2020/04/27/can-estrogen-and-other-sex-hormones-help-men-survive-covid-19/

https://www.nhlbi.nih.gov/science/womens-health-initiative-whi

https://signaturewellness.org/2020/03/15/does-estrogen-protect-women-from-coronavirus/

https://news.yahoo.com/men-high-levels-enzyme-key-022353231.html

https://www.reddit.com/r/COVID19/comments/f3iz3s/ace2_expression_in_kidney_and_testis_may_cause

https://medshadow.org/do-ace-inhibitors-cause-coronavirus/

41

Hormone Receptor Therapy (HRT)

I prefer to look at <u>optimization</u> because hormone levels are going to be different for all patients. This involves taking a personal approach with each individual.

This is the key. How does the organism respond metabolically? That is the goal of treatment. Hormones, metabolism, heart function and stamina, the immune system and body strength. These all equate to a better functioning human body and much more enlightened mental health.

DR LOUISE NEWSON

The figures revealed that there were 9.9 deaths per 100,000 in men compared with 5.5 per 100,000 in women.

Menopause specialist, Dr. Louise Newson today said that specialists are now looking into how hormones could be preventing women from contracting the virus.

Speaking on Good Morning Britain she said: "What we do know is that men have more severe disease with COVID-19 than women and we know that they are more likely to die and more likely to be in intensive care.

"For a while we have been thinking if there is something to do with our hormones, we also know that women who are younger and women who take HRT seem to have some protection."

"We also know pregnancy is protective as well and obviously in pregnancy people have very high hormone levels".

Dr. Louise said she is currently working with Professor Tim Spector and his team with a new app called Zoe.

The app aims to study different COVID symptoms and the team has now started asking questions relating to hormone therapy.

These relate to whether or not a woman is on HRT, whether she is having a period, or if she takes a contraceptive pill.

"We want to find the data so we can obviously provide some evidence for policy makers", Dr. Louise added.

"I'm also working with a team of experts in infectious diseases, clinical pharmacology and public health in Liverpool University so we can really explore this potential role of estrogen in COVID-19

What is HRT?

HRT is a treatment which uses estrogen and progesterone to relieve menopausal symptoms.

As the therapy replaces the hormones that your body is lacking after this change, it's considered to be one of the most effective remedies for the following ailments:

- Hot flashes
- Night sweats
- Reduced sex drive

- Mood swings
- Vaginal dryness

Dr. Louise is presenting hormone replacement therapy for females. Optimal hormone levels in women can improve muscle mass and body composition, improve cholesterol and sugar numbers, help with bone density, and finally improve mood swings and libido. Note is made that the conclusions of the WHI study were flawed. Risk is not increased when bioidentical hormones are used for hormone optimization.

The goal is to move the body back into an optimal hormone balance. We are not talking about giving supra-physiologic doses.

The manner of delivery is important. For women using creams, the half-life is only about eight or 10 hours. Ideally, creams should be used twice a day to maintain even blood levels.

Hormone treatment using pills is more difficult because these are assimilated differently in individuals. With oral medication the first pass after absorption goes to the liver which deactivates about 90% of the oral hormone medication. This makes the oral route more difficult to manage.

For men I prefer a small dose of testosterone given by intramuscular injection twice a week. This levels out the peaks and valleys which can occur if there is a longer interval between injections. Even blood levels improve response. This keeps it from being like a "steroid" program from the gym that presents supra-physiologic doses of hormones.

I prefer injections over pellets, although these seem to work well in some patients who are opposed to taking an injection. When men are on testosterone, I like to

215

give clomiphene (one tablet twice a week) to conserve the feedback loop to the pituitary gland when testosterone is used.

ESTROGEN DOMINANCE

Who can take HRT?

Hormone replacement therapy is widely available to those who are battling menopausal symptoms.

Despite this, the NHS outlines those who may not be suitable for the treatment:

- Patients with a history of breast cancer, ovarian cancer, or cancer of the womb.
- Untreated high blood pressure.
- Someone with liver disease.
- Pregnant patients.
- Patients with a history of blood clots.

"We know that oestrogen is very important for our immunity to the cells that fight any infections and we have oestrogen receptors on these cells."

"We know that stimulating them with oestrogen actually makes them work better, it makes them more efficient so it's more likely to fight the disease."

Numerous theories have emerged as to why men are more likely to have severe cases of the coronavirus.

Evidence shows that men have more angiotensin converting enzymes which allows the virus to enter the lungs and other tissues. Some say testosterone inhibits the immune system. Actually, the opposite is the repair and injury regenerative effect with injury.

In 1991 the Woman's Health Initiative (WHI) Study looked at hormone therapy in many women and demonstrated increased cardiovascular events as well as gynecologic and breast cancer using hormone optimization.

My comment is that the chemicals used in the study were non-bioidentical forms. Hormone therapy also requires monitoring including follow up hormone blood tests. Again, I bring up the concept of a hormone orchestra. Other hormone sections need to be checked as far as overall balance and response even though the sex hormones are the only ones being administered.

Evidence has shown that hormone levels may affect ability for the corona virus to attach to the ACE 2 receptor sites. This can be significant with the current corona pandemic, but it can also be a variable with other future viral infections.

There are no magic bullets. Hormone balance should be optimum to improve cell function, repair, and regeneration. Men also need estrogen and there is balance here with testosterone. Make it a little more complicated by adding progesterone for men.

The treatment regimen is individual and depends on the optimal level for function of the human machine. I am an expert on management and treatment of optimal levels rather than relying on absolute numbers. One of the most important aspects discussing hormone optimization and the coronavirus has to do with overall health promoting resistance and recovery.

Hormone balance should improve cell function for repair and regeneration. This is all about a premature drop in hormone levels. Chemical and hormone balance is a key initial step for healing. Hormones promote resistance to infection. Cholesterol and sugar metabolism improve. It provides protection from cancer and protects from degenerative chronic physical conditions.

Progesterone is another aspect of this balance that has been relatively ignored by conventional medicine in both men and women.

VITAMIN D - THIS IS A HORMONE

The other thing to bring up is vitamin D. The chemical structure of vitamin D is a steroid ring. This is similar to estrogen and testosterone. Cholesterol also has a steroid ring for a chemical structure and is the precursor for formation of vitamin D.

Vitamin D3 serves as a hormone and is used in the overall balance of sex hormones. I do not think that this is traditionally recognized but a smoother optimization with hormones occurs in patients when vitamin D levels are raised. The effect of the other hormones improves. I advise my patients to take their vitamin D at bedtime. The usual dose for many of my patients is 10,000 units per night. I have seen no toxicity with vitamin D the past 20 years. If the vitamin D is taken at bedtime it can initiate a better sleep cycle. This lowers cortisol and may improve growth hormone naturally.

I have had several patients in their mid-20s with very low testosterone levels. These would not come up except with extremely high doses of testosterone that would normally be considered supra physiologic doses. Sometimes even these did not consistently raise their serum testosterone levels. The vitamin D levels were also in the gutter. When vitamin D was replaced the amount of testosterone needed for hormone optimization decreased.

The conversion of vitamin D2 to active D3 can be inhibited by preservatives in processed food. One of the chief ones is sodium benzoate. So, I have patients that live in the sun and still have low vitamin D levels that need supplementation.

There is a hormone orchestra made up of various hormone sections. Improving function in one section allows the other sections as well as the overall orchestra to play better. Cortisol is another hormone that needs to be considered as far as overall balance. I will commonly give a short course of growth hormone to help the patient recover from an injury and initiate repair. Sometimes this is used for a short course during wound healing and recovery.

Thymic hormones are another component that is not really appreciated by conventional medicine. The thymus gland is small and located in the upper chest a few inches below the thyroid gland at the base of the neck. It provides an immune function, particularly to stimulate T cells, which are the ones that defend against the virus and other invaders. There is a peptide that can be given intermittently that may be effective during an epidemic. This is thymosin alpha-1 which stimulates activity of the thymus gland and improves immune function. Another is TB 500. I have had several patients who took this as a preventive for coronavirus. Several told me about thickening of hair with the TB 500.

Are there any clinical studies? No. I am giving you a personal observation. This is what I do and how I learn.

The bottom line is that there is no cookbook for everyone. I spend enough time with each patient looking at the metabolic status and ability to heal and try to optimize their results.

LOW TESTERONE IS NOT HEALTHY

- Basically, the key is to stay ahead of the premature drop in hormones that is the result of environmental influences.
- This is the ballgame for good overall health and quality longevity. Testosterone is only one inning.
- As a physician, I am the patient's coach. That is what I do.

This recent article Low Testosterone Can Lead to Early Death emphasizes the importance of maintaining optimal hormone levels. The most important factor in the **Danish study** indicates that the patients with the greatest 10-year decline in testosterone had the worst prognosis as far as survival.

What does this mean? I am 70 years old and the average testosterone levels in guys my age is 40% below those of an age matched group back in the 1950's. The environment is causing premature drop in hormones. Hormone Disruptors, so we are told to accept "that you are just getting older" instead of "what can I do to make myself better."

Optimization of hormones provides good physiologic function of the human machine. This not only improves longevity but the patient benefits from an increased quality of life. As in maintenance of an automobile, choices in fuel source may change function. And the body has things like the motor as well as cooling and electrical systems.

Sometimes a new engine part or body repair is needed. Optimization is repair and maintenance.

Before initiating a program, a detailed workup is essential and includes testing that provides data not commonly seen with usual conventional medicine physical examinations. This includes comprehensive blood work including testing not routinely obtained. It is important to start with a good medical baseline to give a roadmap to direct where a program should go.

Following that, hormone optimization can be approached using supplements or many times hormones with an emphasis on bioidentical hormones.

Look at this example:

A middle-age man (50) comes in with a little bit of a paunch and is asked about his medical health. He states it is pretty good. He goes to the gym. He tries to eat right. As far as medication, he takes something for cholesterol, another for blood pressure, a heart pill, and something for sugar. Oh, and Viagra certainly helps. His doctor told him that all his numbers were under control (whatever that means).

I ask you—-is this **truly healthy?** Is there a balance (chemical and hormonal) for the "human machine" to function optimally?

Digest this comment.

Cholesterol *is an essential item for health. Besides providing structure of individual cell walls it serves as a precursor for neurotransmitters in the brain. Cholesterol is used by the body to make sex hormones and vitamin D (and YES vitamin D is a hormone). Suboptimal hormones lead to an increase in the blood cholesterol levels. Rather than throwing a pill at the cholesterol it is more appropriate to improve chemical and hormone balance.*

221

Focusing on more optimum physiologic function of the human machine will lead to long-term and good quality health.

*As far as adult onset or type II diabetes and **sugar metabolism**, this also is definitely adversely affected by suboptimal testosterone. Instead of blood sugar pills and insulin, optimal testosterone levels could bring blood sugars down into an acceptable range without medication.*

*So, the patient above could be **treated piece by piece** as far as conventional medicine - a pill is given for such and such number and another pill for something else.*

A step further is to consider the entire human machine, specifically looking at overall physiologic function at the cellular and metabolic level. A program is based on the initial workup. After that, appropriate monitoring at intervals for patients receiving hormone optimization is essential.

Basically, the key is to stay ahead of the premature drop in hormones that is the result of environmental influences.

This is the ballgame for good overall health and quality longevity. Testosterone is only one inning. Think about rebooting cells in your body that have depleted some vital chemicals in the body.

Again, I am the patient's coach. That is what I do.

https://growyouthful.com/remedy/progesterone.php

https://www.progesteronetherapy.com/progesterone-for-men.html

https://www.linkedin.com/pulse/unique-aspects-vitamin-d-joseph-edward-bosiljevac-jr-md-phd-facs/?trackingId=Yl87UiYq9V https://www.wsj.com/articles/vitamin-d-and-coronavirus-disparities-11587078141

42

An Apocalyptic Virus

HEALTH ISSUES MAKE US THINK

- Avian flu—bird flu.
- Chicken farming will kill us.
- Remember the advertisement of the cow writing on the sign - *Eat More Chicken.*
- Survival of the fittest.

As a clinician I look at resistance and recovery from any infectious agent. The world is in this second stage now. Where do we go from here?

Bill Gates gave a seminar in 2015 which some today feel relates to the current pandemic.

Apocalypse means the big one. Lethality. That is not quite what COVID-19 has been. It has been more of an attack from within, one that takes away our humanity while dividing us as a people. No. The bad one is the avian flu. Bird flu.

The avian flu is zoonotic. This means the virus can spread between animals and humans. The coronavirus is zoonotic and spread by bats. Other examples of zoonotic diseases are tuberculosis, measles, and whooping cough.

How many chickens do we eat each year? How about eggs? I will not get into any detail on the crowded and miserable lifestyle of these animals. That is our food source. Do sweatshop eggs and chickens pose a problem to our personal health? This and any other source of food that we intake as nutrition certainly has an effect on our ability to take on viruses and the world we live in.

In the past I had many patients say that they were instructed to avoid red meat, so they had been eating a lot of chicken. It is not necessarily the red meat but the food source. If the meat is grass fed, healthy, and raised humanely then it is better for us to ingest. How about those darn chickens? Honestly the system for raising our own food is highly questionable at times.

Another example of the lifestyle is establishment of pig and cattle farms. It is easy for contamination and the zoonotic coronavirus goes from bat to our food supply.

The Spanish flu in 1918 hit primarily 20 to 34-year-olds as far as fatalities. That was an Avian or bird flu.

With the current pandemic I am trying to learn more about biology, resistance, and recovery. As a teacher I preach to take care of yourself. Longevity requires some discipline. Make the body ready to resist infection, heal, and repair itself. That is my suggestion as far as an apocalyptic virus. Survival of the fittest. Look at personal maintenance.

Apocalyptic? There is evidence suggesting that the current coronavirus was genetically developed by the Chinese government.

Be that as it may, the situation here is for us to learn as

a society to deal with a pandemic. There could be a worse virus that pops up from any other part of the world. It means we still do not have all the answers. No magic bullets. <u>Personal health is a big key</u>.

https://www.linkedin.com/pulse/what-does-mean-reboot-joseph-edward-bosiljevac-jr-md-phd-facs/

https://www.news.com.au/lifestyle/health/health-problems/chicken-farming-could-lead-to-apocalyptic-virus-worse-than-coronavirus/news-story/63c87b51da43fd54a76405c8ca279016

https://www.linkedin.com/pulse/personal-maintenance-reversibility-bosiljevac-jr-md-phd-facs/?trackingId=1UPb%2F%2BUynansYf3R2REz2A%3D%3D

https://www.foxnews.com/world/chinese-virologist-coronavirus-cover-up-flee-hong-kong-whistleblower

43

Immunity and Resistance

New York City is starting to reopen after a lockdown. This was more long-standing in the epicenter than other parts of the country. The primary difference is the population density.

Monday, June 22 was phase 2 in Manhattan with restaurants serving outdoors and barbershops and spas opening.

The Big Apple's not-so-grand reopening: NYC eases out of lockdown - but Manhattan stores like Saks Fifth Avenue remain boarded up with barbed wire protected by security guards with dogs after a week of riots and looting.

Phase 1 of NYC's reopening began Monday, June 8 bringing between 200,000 and 400,000 persons back to work.

THE CITY SPEEDING UP

- The biggest change is in retail - all retailers can now reopen but must provide curbside pick-up services only.
- Some are hesitant to get back to work because workers fear they will contract the virus.

- Masks and hand sanitizer are being given out for free on the subway to try to calm people's fears.
- The reality in NYC on Monday is that many stores have boarded up their windows for fear of being looted.
- Other industries that resume on Monday are manufacturing and construction, but the biggest difference in the Big Apple will be stores being allowed to reopen again.
- The next phase is to allow outdoor dining at restaurants with hair salons and offices to reopen, but that is not expected to begin until July.
- It remains unclear if and when indoor dining or indoor bar service will resume, and gyms remain closed.
- Movie theaters and other entertainment services are in the final phase - a date has not been announced.
- The subway remained open throughout the pandemic but on a reduced service - as of Monday, it is operating at 95 percent of its usual service.
- De Blasio announced five more bus routes that will be put in place between June and October.

Study: COVID-19 Much Deadlier Than Flu; 1.3% Death Rate among Symptomatic Patients.

- Researchers say if same number of Americans contract coronavirus by the end of 2020 as those who catch the flu, as many as 500,000 people will die.
- Conservative estimate of 20% of population infected would mean anywhere from 350,000 to 1.2M deaths by year's end.

20 June 2020

- Cuomo threatens 14-day quarantine for anyone who travels to New York from states where coronavirus cases are rising.
- New York has flattened its curve so much that only 0.9 percent of the tests being done every day are coming back positive.
- On Wednesday, of the more than 60,000 people tested statewide, 618 were positive.
- Total COVID hospitalizations in NY are down to 1,400 - at their worst the number was more than 18,000.
- Now, Cuomo wants to avoid people in states where it is rising to visit NY where it may trigger a second wave.
- New York had the longest and harshest lockdown whereas other states were more relaxed.
- In Texas, Florida and Arizona, cases and hospitalizations are rising quickly.

AN UNEVEN PLAYING FIELD

Florida, Arizona and Texas all experience COVID-19 infection spikes but death rates fall across the nation amid hope the virus may finally be weakening its grip after killing more than 120,000 Americans.

- Florida, Arizona, Texas and California are among the states that continue to have record spikes in daily coronavirus infections.
- The number of daily deaths, however, now appears to be gradually declining in those states.

- More than 120,000 Americans have now died of COVID-19 and 2.2 million have been infected. That is 1% of the population overall that have been infected.
- Health experts, however, warn deaths could spike again because the death rate often lags several weeks behind the infection rate.
- Experts say the fact that younger people are now accounting for a large number of the new cases could also have an impact in several weeks.
- Young people could currently be infecting their elderly relatives and other at-risk people, which could drive up hospitalizations and deaths.
- Health officials say the upward trends in testing positivity rates that several states are reporting is particularly alarming.
- The World Health Organization considers positivity rates above 5% to be especially concerning.
- Florida, Texas, Arizona and South Carolina have positive rates above 10%.

The big deal is asymptomatic carriers. If you have symptoms the incidence is higher for transmitting the virus.

Only 37% of New Yorkers who think they've had coronavirus have antibodies to prove it, testing of more than 1,300 citizens. As I review this before publication a month after originally written, more extensive testing shows overall 1 % of the general population carry antibodies.

We will talk later about the complex immune picture that occurs with this and other viruses.

Study: Initial U.S. COVID-19 infection rate may be 80

times greater than believed

- There may be some cross immunity from other infections.

People who have had suffered from a COLD in the past could be protected against COVID-19.

Scientists analyzed 11 blood samples from people more than two years ago. At least half the blood samples had T cells that recognized SARS-CoV-2

Some 20 per cent had T cells, which are immune cells that would be able to kill it.

The researchers said it was 'tempting to speculate' those people would be protected from severe COVID-19. But this remains to be proven.

BEIJING (Reuters) - A Beijing district put itself on a "wartime" footing and the capital banned tourism and sports events on Saturday after a cluster of novel coronavirus infections centered around a major wholesale market sparked fears of a new wave of COVID-19.

The entire Xinfadi market was shut down at 3 a.m. on Saturday (1900 GMT on Friday), after two men working at a meat research centre who had recently visited the market were reported to have the virus. It was not immediately clear how they had been infected.

The bottom line is social distancing and personal hygiene with masks, gloves, and frequent washing of hands.

Breathing or talking may be the most common ways coronavirus is spread - and contaminated surfaces only play a small role, according to Chinese scientists

- Study found COVID patients exhale millions of viral particles per hour while breathing.
- Suggests breathing and talking main source of transmission along with coughs.
- Scientists said people were unlikely to catch viruses from contaminated surfaces.

AN INFORMATION TREADMILL

The WHO walks backs its claim that the spread of coronavirus by asymptomatic people is 'very rare' as Harvard scientists slam the organization for 'creating confusion' and say those with no symptoms ARE spreaders.

- On Monday, the WHO said it's very rare that asymptomatic people spread coronavirus and that they are not a 'main driver' of new infection.
- The UN health agency said this is based on new evidence from countries that are doing detailed contact tracing.
- Harvard's Global Health institute says the WHO 'created confusion' with its statement that those without symptoms are not readily spreading the virus.
- Scientists from the Institute say because asymptomatic patients are transmitting the virus, people still need to socially distance and wear masks.
- On Tuesday, the WHO walked back its comments and said that its assertion that asymptomatic spread is 'rare' is a misunderstanding.

CORONA 101

What is the risk of eating out? What precautions are helpful?

- Are you or anyone you live with over age 65 or at risk of severe illness? The risk of getting a serious infection from COVID-19 increases with age and certain medical conditions.
- Do you and those you will be interacting with follow the same steps to prevent infection, such as wearing masks and washing hands?
- Can you maintain 6 feet of social distance in a reasonable way?
- How often will you need to share items? Sharing isn't caring during a pandemic. As a rule, don't share items. But if you must, are you (or the restaurant) properly cleaning and disinfecting them between each use?
- What's the current level of COVID-19 spread in your community? "The lower the level of community transmission, the safer it is for you to go out."

A PERSONAL MEASURE WORTH TRYING

The British developed the use of iodine - inexpensive, effective, and convenient.

PVP-1 (Betadine) is a good general disinfectant and has good antiviral qualities. It can be applied to mucous membranes inside the nose or mouth, which is where the virus collects. Viral content was measured in healthcare providers as well as patients during the general hospital care for COVID patients. Mucous samples for viruses were taken frequently when there was exposure to the **oropharyngeal** tract such as intubation.

- First of all, it is safe for the nose and mouth with proper dilution. Exposure to iodine during this study was well within previously recorded safe levels.
- Second, it significantly reduces the viral load on surfaces where droplets from sneezing and touching the mouth are encountered.
- Third, it was shown the effect can last for three hours.
- Get a small bottle of normal saline (0.9% sodium chloride) nasal spray from the pharmacy. Use 2/3 the contents of this bottle and add 1/3 volume with the standard Betadine solution. That is your dilution. As mentioned, it appears an application lasts for three hours. It can be sprayed into the nasal passages as well as the mouth. As far as the mouth application, wait one minute or so before any water or anything else is ingested afterward.
- This is another example of something learned from experience with this pandemic. The use of a Betadine type spray in the nose and mouth is so effective, convenient, and inexpensive. A simple way to improve hygiene as part of our lifestyle. It can be used for high exposure situations. However, for the United Kingdom health workers it was used every three hours during their working shift.

I have an oral surgeon colleague and when I mentioned this to Dr. Charlie Kaner, he explained their office is way in front using an iodine solution. His particular product does not cause staining of teeth or tongue. My time as a patient with Dr. K reinforces my appreciation of his experience. I am still alive trying to keep teeth going another 50 years.

Iodine mouthwash could protect against COVID-19 and reduce the viral load of infected patients because it has 'significant' virus-killing ability when used on sister viruses SARS and MERS, scientists claim.

Researchers said that specific types of mouthwash - made with the chemicals povidone and iodine - can have 'significant virucidal activity.'

Iodine mouthwash is stronger than popular shop-bought products such as Listerine or Colgate, which typically don't contain the antiseptic chemical - it is more commonly used by dentists. One brand that contains iodine is Betadine.

The following article talks about the spread when people are out doing "healthful" exercises. Thirty feet is a wide distance.

For example, asymptomatic coronavirus transmission appears worse than SARS or influenza — a runner can leave a 'slipstream' of 30 feet.

There may be some cross immunity from other infections. Viruses are always mutating, but can be similar to others we have seen in the past. People who have suffered from a COLD in the past could be protected against COVID-19.

And there is a rare case where a woman from Texas was infected with the COVID-19 virus a second time. This is probably on the basis of an altered immune system response where she had not formed preventive antibodies and her underlying immune system allowed her to get sick again.

The virus appears to be adapting to people. The so-called spikes of the corona structure may become more numerous. These are what latch them to the lining of the human nose and throat.

There are many variables and here are various scenarios:

- The human organism is resistant to COVID-19 and the virus never takes hold. This is the best case ever!
- The human organism is resistant to COVID-19 because it has been affected with the SARS Coronavirus or H3N3 (which is an avian or bird flu virus) and effective related antibodies are present.
- An infection develops and COVID-19 antibodies form for future resistance.
- The immune system is sick and is not able to form antibodies even after an active infection.
- There is no black and white answer. Many people want immediate information, assistance, and no mistakes. It is a very demanding situation from many angles.

So there is a personal aspect outside of a cookbook. A lot of current research teaches us more about the virus. There are two viruses. There is the coronavirus which is also related to the SARS and the MERS virus. Then we have the avian or bird flu viruses such as H3N2 and H3 N3. These are cousins and really should not react as far as antigenic or immune properties. However, there is a big question whether exposure to these improve resistance with further corona or avian flu infections.

As far as infection, symptoms may be absent, minimal, severe, and 1-2% fatal. Overall incidence is 1% of population at this time.

Occasionally a strong defensive attack may be serious. Sometimes a patient can have an overwhelming illness that may be due to an active immune system. Look at this case:

So, there is a growing body of evidence that at least some of the problems caused by SARS-CoV-2 are the result of how the virus manipulates the immune system in order to maintain an infection. How much of the COVID-19 symptoms it explains isn't clear yet, nor is it obvious whether the variability of symptoms is a result of patient-specific immune responses. But in light of this growing body of evidence, it's a safe bet that researchers will be working hard to find out.

Again, a virus can affect the human being and the body is strong enough to fight this off without becoming infected. Antibodies may not form in this situation. Sometimes a mild infection will occur and antibodies will form. Sometimes a severe illness will occur and antibodies form. If the patient's immune system is down, the patient could become infected and not form appropriate antibodies.

There is ultraviolet wavelength light now available to sterilize masks and other personal supplies. There has been discussion of these lights used in high traffic areas such as subways and airports.

More extensive long-term use of masks may prevent the second wave, although how long can Americans be expected to wear masks? Months? Years? Widespread face mask use could control a second wave of COVID-19. Personal health measures seem much more likely and manageable for a long term answer. Masks are probably the most significant preventive factor.

The British developed the use of iodine - inexpensive, effective, and convenient. PVP-1(Betadine) is a good general disinfectant and has good antiviral qualities. The health workers use this nose spray on the job.

Cultural hygiene plays a part as far as re-entry.

All cultures have two primary desires - safety and freedom. In other words, keep me safe but leave me alone. Social changes will be looked at as far as the current epidemic. Here in New York City many immigrant families live with numerous generations living in a small household.

Looking at infectivity there are several variabilities and variants involved. Who can fight infection? Why is there more prevalent risk in some groups? Variance with individuals is not all genetic.

Genetics - Asians are likely to have more resistance because of frequent exposure to many viruses that started in Asia, particularly the avian bird flu and the coronavirus. There are a lot of open markets in Asia that allow these viruses to pass from animal to human (zoonotic virus).

There continue to be more reports about the innate difference in blood types fighting this infection. Type O is better than other types in this case with corona, but also with cardiovascular diseases and cancer.

There is always a combination genetic and lifestyle component:

- Some NYC neighborhoods have seen death rates from coronavirus nearly 15 times higher than others.
- The pandemic has revealed wide disparities in how people have been affected.
- Starrett City in East New York, Brooklyn has the highest death rate in the city.
- Far Rockaway and Flushing in Queens, followed by a

section of the northeast Bronx, and Coney Island in Brooklyn have also been badly affected.

- Only the Financial District in Lower Manhattan has recorded zero deaths.
- At least 190,000 cases of coronavirus have been reported in NYC by the end of June. In total there have been more than 15,900 confirmed deaths and a further 4,800 probable deaths.

Region - the geographical area and climate may suppress the virus or it mutates and becomes more variable. Infection can relate to population density and lifestyle.

Also, mid day sunlight is capable of inactivating 90 percent or more of the SARS-CoV-19 virus after 34 minutes of exposure.

Lifestyle - some nations did not shut down completely like New York City. Our North American society may be more susceptible because of the lack of prior contact with Asian viruses. There may also be some subtle aspects about overall health that decrease the resistance to infection and also recovery. Americans tend to be on the unhealthy side compared to the rest of the world.

Americans are not used to wearing a mask. I live in the epicenter of this pandemic in the middle of Manhattan. The population density here may be 10,000 persons per block in the upper east side, Manhattan.

At the peak of the epidemic masks and personal hygiene are important. It is necessary to isolate high risk patients. And, go back to getting your machine rebooted. This can improve your overall metabolic function and immune system.

What many do not appreciate is the important aspect of personal health. Changes in health can be very subtle in society and it is accepted that by aging into the mid 80's your life will be over.

https://www.linkedin.com/pulse/can-you-get-younger-joseph-edward-bosiljevac-jr-md-phd-facs/?trackingId=YpvD-sqqJ80moEutzbWJdzg%3D%3D

https://www.linkedin.com/pulse/benefit-rejuvenation-joseph-edward-bosiljevac-jr-md-phd-facs-1f/?trackingId=Y7x9O8C1DIJEd0Uuemqg%3D%3D

https://www.studyfinds.org/study-covid-19-much-deadlier-than-flu-1-3-death-rate-among-symptomatic-patients/

https://www.studyfinds.org/study-initial-u-s-covid-19-infection-rate-may-be-80-times-greater-han-believed/

https://www.reuters.com/article/us-health-coronavirus-beijing/beijing-district-in-wartime-emergency-after-virus-cluster-at-major-food-market-idUSKBN23K03V

https://www.linkedin.com/pulse/16-april-i-came-across-release-from-british-group-joseph-edward/?trackingId=%2Fi40yYXC

https://canoe.com/news/world/i-was-floored-texas-woman-gets-covid-19-for-a-second-time

https://arstechnica.com/science/2020/05/a-look-at-what-covid-patients-are-telling-us-about-the-virus-and-risks/

44

Comparisons and Similarities

Father's Day, 21 June 2020

- Cardinal Dolan speaks on TV about social healing.
- The city is busier with people outside. Masks are being worn by most.
- City traffic is almost normal during the week.
- With the concern over the risk of infection and use of the subway, there are more people driving.
- Restaurants open with outdoor tables tomorrow. I passed by some tonight.
- New York has a ways to go but I see a good start!!
- Trump has a limited open event in Tulsa. Politics continue.

22 June 2020

- Phase 2 opens businesses and outside eating in restaurants. Spas and barbershops will have limited activity.
- I need a haircut—four months now. I made an appoint-

ment for tomorrow.

- Some reports are coming in stating an increasing incidence in new cases. This has not been resolved. We are still in this epidemic, which is reasonably controlled at this time.

25 June 2020

- Overall national cases continue to increase last week. Florida, California, and Texas are the worst areas for infection at this point.
- NY governor Cuomo wants to control patients arriving in NYC from areas reporting increased incidence of disease, like Florida, Texas, and California.

At this point we had been through a lockdown of businesses and quarantined at home. Only until recently have we started the reopening phase of the economy.

NOT UNLIKE OUR PAST

I compare this to this to an epidemic from 50 years ago. Take a look at this paper (see link at end of chapter) on Woodstock, the original one back in 1969. The Hong Kong Flu raged through America as major events went ahead with participation and fanfare.

This Woodstock article is very interesting. There was no social distancing. Hundreds of thousands crowded into a small space. The economy was not shut down.

How did a 'filthy' Woodstock still go ahead during the 1968 Hong Kong flu pandemic that killed 100,000 Americans and infected everyone from President Lyndon Johnson to the Apollo 8 crew? It even infected SeaWorld's famous Shamu, the killer whale.

Astronaut Frank Borman vomited repeatedly on his trip to the moon due to having the flu.

The 1968 Hong Kong flu pandemic (caused by the H3N2 virus) killed 100,000 Americans and 1 million people world-wide. The virus was spread in the US by troops returning home from the Vietnam War.

More Americans died from the Hong Kong flu pandemic than the combined number of US casualties in the Vietnam and Korean Wars. It also killed so many people in Berlin that corpses were stored in subway tunnels.

As of today (June 2020), H3N2 was deadlier than COVID-19 which has a current world wise death toll of 315,000, though it is expected to surpass the number of those killed during the 1968 pandemic.

Both Tallulah Bankhead and CIA Director, Allen Dulles died of the Hong Kong Flu.

The Hong Kong flu pandemic raged on through early 1970 without any government mandated closures, stay-at-home orders and restrictions on public gatherings.

NYC declared a state of emergency but kept schools and businesses open - 400,000 people attended Woodstock in 1969 and festival organizer Joel Rosenman said, 'there were no containment measures to defy.' The virus ran its course.

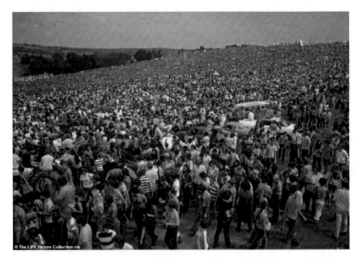

3 Days of Peace and Music.

Amid growing outrage over state closures, some experts say that the 1968 pandemic puts the current COVID-19 shutdowns into perspective.

The H3N2 virus still exists today and re-surfaces during flu season every year.

Consider this paper (see link at end of chapter) published by Tate Delloye in May of 2020. Many Americans are wondering why we are treating this pandemic so differently and with so much damage to the small businesses in our country. We have seen sickness before that did not halt the economy as we did this time around.

They lived on top of each other. Restaurants were not closed, and neither were stores. Just look at this as compared to the current coronavirus pandemic.

I am not being critical of how it is has been handled.

Certainly the mortality rate might have been much higher since the coronavirus appears to be more contagious than the usual bird flu virus. So, the social measures of personal hygiene continue to be very important.

Within two weeks of the initial outbreak in July 1968, 500,000 people in Hong Kong came down with the flu which caused upper respiratory infection, chills, fever, muscle pain and weakness. It was brought to the US via returning soldiers coming home from the Vietnam War and by December all 50 states were infected with the H3N2 virus.

The New York Times said the flu was 'one of the worst in the nation's history' and as it neared its peak in December 1968, the City Health Commissioner estimated that one in every five New Yorkers would end up contracting the illness. 'This is just the beginning, the worst is yet to come,' said a doctor for the city health department.

Hospitals were overrun and those who were infected were sent home and told to rest. 'In the meantime, they can take aspirin, tea, lemon drinks, whisky or brandy according to taste,' said a Hong Kong official to journalists.

Severely ill patients were put on ventilators, often without any improvement. New York City's blood bank was depleted, which forced hospitals to cancel both elective and life-saving surgeries. Absenteeism in the workplace was up 50% in the United States, garbage collectors in West Germany had to bury bodies because the undertakers couldn't keep up with the demand, while corpses in Berlin had to be stored in subway tunnels.

Though unlike the restrictive measures taken today, there were no stay-at-home orders, harsh lockdown rules and state-wide closures. People still went to work, students attended school, Broadway theaters stayed open and 75,000 spectators watched the New York Jets play in Super Bowl III.

Now consider this paper written by Gail Dutton, published on April 13, 2020. **The 1968 Pandemic Strain (H3N2) Persists. Will COVID-19?**

1968 was a bad year for the flu but, as pandemics go, it was pretty mild. Scientists called the flu strain that hit the world H3N2. It's still around.

Globally, about one million people died until the outbreak faded during the winter of 1969-70. In the U.S., the death toll was approximately 100,000 – three or four times the average annual death toll for flu since 2010, according to CDC figures. Most of those deaths were among people aged 65 or older.

Although the COVID-19 death toll has not yet reached the numbers of H3N2, it still continues to climb. According to Johns Hopkins University's continually updated Coronavirus Resource Center, U.S. deaths for COVID-19 are now in excess of 116,000, and New York has seen over 22,000. (July of 2020). August 9, 2020 U.S. death rate is 163,000 and New York 33,000.

The H3N2 flu originated in Hong Kong in July of 1968 and appeared in the U.S. in September and is still circulating as a type of Influenza A. H3N2 was present among the 2019 flu strains and in the swine flu outbreak earlier in the decade.

Like so many viruses implicated in 20th century pandemics, both the H3N2 virus and the SARS-Cov-2 virus that causes COVID-19 exhibited cross-species transmission, appearing first in animals before jumping to humans and, sometimes, back to animals. A canine outbreak occurred in late 2017 in Ontario, Canada and persisted until October 2018.

H3N2 is considered one of the most troubling flu strains because, like COVID-19, it is highly contagious. And zoonotic—can spread from animals to humans.

Because H3N2 was closely related to the 1957 pandemic, many people were immune. This kept the 1968 H3N2 flu epidemic relatively mild, especially when compared to the 1918 Spanish flu. For some reason, however – possibly antigenic drift – the second wave of the H3N2 flu that struck in 1969 was more deadly.

Differences in immunity are evident as the virus mutated during its global spread, as shown by the different patterns of infection and death.

Edwin D. Kilbourne, (since deceased) professor of microbiology and immunology at New York Medical College, in a 2006 article comparing the influenza pandemics of the 20th century, found that outbreaks in Japan were small and scattered. Western Europe, including the United Kingdom, experienced increased illnesses but no increased death rates during the first year of the pandemic. The U.S., however, experienced high illness and death rates the first year, beginning on the West Coast where the virus was first introduced.

"Researchers speculated that (H3N2's) more sporadic and variable impact in different regions of the world were mediated by differences in prior N2 immunity. Therefore, the 1968 pandemic has been aptly characterized as 'smoldering,'" Kilbourne wrote. Emphasizing that point, vaccination by Air Force cadets with the H2N2 vaccine reduced H3N2 infections by 54%.

HOW HAVE OTHER COUNTRIES HANDLED THE PANDEMIC?

Hong Kong managed to contain the COVID-19 epidemic without totally locking out. Measures were taken that developed because of interval exposure to the bird flu. Closing schools was a big part as far as the social distancing. Large group public social events were canceled.

In the most recent (March) survey, 85 percent of respondents reported avoiding crowded places, and 99 percent reported wearing face masks when leaving home — up from 75 per cent and 61 per cent respectively from the first survey in January.

Americans are not used to wearing masks.

Vietnam was another country that avoided a large catastrophe by acting early when a Chinese retired man living in Vietnam and his father came back from Wuhan and presented as the first cases. After January 23 all flights from Wuhan were canceled. Contact tracing to direct quarantine was a priority. 43% of patients that were positive with antibodies had been asymptomatic. Appropriate measures were taken at airports and by late March nobody could get in the country.

This highlights the effects of the contact tracing and quarantine. On the 1st of February a national epidemic was announced. There was a directed lockdown for elderly and disabled patients. They went through a routine that has been thought out and performed before. Acting early, safer, and smarter. This was all in response to their experience in the past.

Tracing was a big deal where relatives and friends can

be called and anyone with possible contact going into focal quarantine. The more I think about this, it is so simple. A directed focal quarantine.

The same occurred with South Korea.

Japan had a low infection rate. Some of this may be natural immunity from exposure to many Corona and bird flu viruses in the past. It is natural for them to use masks and gloves routinely or whenever increased risk is present.

Japan's state of emergency ended when new cases of the coronavirus dwindled to mere dozens. It got there despite largely ignoring the default playbook.

No restrictions were placed on residents' movements, and businesses from restaurants to hairdressers stayed open. No high-tech apps that tracked people's movements were deployed. The country doesn't have a center for disease control. And even as nations were exhorted to "test, test, test," Japan has tested just 0.2% of its population - one of the lowest rates among developed countries. Not a lot of testing.

The early response was also boosted by an unlikely happening. Japan's battle with the virus first came to mainstream international attention with its much-criticized response to the Diamond Princess cruise ship in February.

Another example is that of New Zealand. The first case of coronavirus was on February 28. This was a month after the first case documented in the United States. On March 14 when six cases had been confirmed Prime Minister Jacinda Ardern announced immediate self-isolation for two weeks for anyone entering the country. Foreign nationals were banned from entering the country on March 20. On March 23 a level of lockdown was initiated.

The end of March more severe levels of isolation were initiated and through April order restrictions were tightened considerably.

New Zealand has a population of 5 million people. Approximately 1500 contracted the disease and 22 died.

In early June a stretch of 17 days had passed with no new cases reported. Almost all restrictions were lifted.

Now in August a few isolated cases were identified following birthday parties and funeral gatherings. Also, a case was from a patient who flew in from Pakistan.

Eliminating the virus will not end the economic pain or any of loss of jobs. The tourism industry is particularly hard hit.

At the peak of the epidemic masks and personal hygiene are important. It is necessary to isolate high risk patients. And go back to getting your machine rebooted. This can improve your overall metabolic function and immune system.

People who have had suffered from a COLD in the past could be protected against COVID-19, scientists claim

Scientists analyzed 11 blood samples from people more than two years ago. At least half the blood samples had T cells that recognized SARS-CoV-2

Some 20 per cent had T cells, which are immune cells that would be able to kill it.

The researchers said it was 'tempting to speculate' those people would be protected from severe COVID-19. But this remains to be proven. There may be some cross immunity from other infections, even the common cold. This has also been shown with MMR vaccination.

https://www.dailymail.co.uk/sciencetech/article-8439609/MMR-jab-used-prevent-measles-mumps-rubella-help-protect-against-COVID-19.html

https://www.dailymail.co.uk/news/article-8320761/Woodstock-occurred-Hong-Kong-flu-pandemic-killed-1-million-people-worldwide-100-000-Americans.html

https://www.cnn.com/2020/05/29/asia/coronavirus-vietnam-intl-hnk/index.html

https://www.bloomberg.com/news/articles/2020-05-22/did-japan-just-beat-the-virus-without-lockdowns-or-mass-testing

45

Truly Move Ahead, Focusing on Yourself

Practicing age management in New York City the last 12 years, I quickly found that getting older means body parts wear out. Working with retired NFL and NBA players I began doing stem cell treatment for joint and soft tissue injuries. Then I started treating military Special Forces members. With this group I began dealing with other conditions such as traumatic brain injury, MS, emphysema, autoimmune disorders, and liver problems as well as regeneration from various soft tissue and joint injuries. Look at the entire human machine, not just a body part. The human body wants to heal itself.

Basically, the philosophy is rebooting cells to work normally. Peptides play a part. In addition, so is the use of biologically active NAD, exosomes, and stem cells. These will be discussed in more detail in Part 4 of this book, but the idea is simple. Regeneration leads to rejuvenation. Rejuvenated cells function more optimally. Rebooting cells is more than just an oil change. This is an overhaul.

Personal maintenance is so important. We take care of our autos, riding lawn mower, golf cart, and other things better than our health. Again, I state overhaul or oil change? That is what I offer my patients. Unique personal plans are developed with my wide background and experience.

Variance with individuals is not all genetic. There may be some difference between genetic groups or perhaps related to geography, lifestyle, prior exposure to these viruses, and overall health. Also, recall there's a coronavirus and a cousin which is a bird flu that causes the typical flu infection. All of these things have a mixed picture. This is not black-and-white. Problem-solving is part of what attracted me to medicine.

What is the result of this rebooting?

1. If you are 50 years of age (actually 40 may be more realistic) recognize that certain biological chemicals in your cells have decreased and may even be significantly depleted. The rejuvenation program will restore cells to function more optimally. Chemical and hormone balance can be evaluated. This rejuvenation program consists of intravenous NAD, exosomes, stem cells, the use of a peptide, and possible other treatments. This program will renew your system to function at a biologically younger age.

2. Even if you consider yourself in good health, subtle aging changes have been going on. Some of these can be reversed by going through a rejuvenation program.

3. For patients with a chronic condition or autoimmune disease there may be multiple symptoms. These patients will be sent to multiple specialists and receive

various treatments. If this patient would go through a rejuvenation program to reboot cells to function optimally then many symptoms would abate. This would leave a more defined program for recovery and fewer specialists. Multiple specialists never look at the entire picture.

Then we get to the point of immunity. What determines that? The immune system is important. But I narrow it down and just mention this as personal health.

Personal maintenance is important. We have talked about rebooting cells so they function normally. As you get older, a rejuvenation program is important to restore body function to an optimum range.

Reboot means to restore chemical balance inside the cell so that it functions normally. Think in terms of the construction of a building. There is a solid foundation and then the different building materials. Each needs to provide support. Consider each of these materials as body cells. The cells need energy to support the human machine. Rebooting cells restores cell energy and function. With an appropriate program I can see 120 quality years as a lifespan.

Rebooting cells is the best approach to improve personal health. 90% of our society does not understand what it means to reboot. As we get older, basic biological chemicals in the cells wear down.

Subtle things occur and society accepts that you are just getting older. However this may be premature and just not understood or expected.

If cells do not function well, degeneration occurs in the body. Society accepts this as normal aging. However, it can also be reversed and restored. Oil change or an overhaul?

Look at the summary of the patient noted in this case review:

There is a 48-year-old retired Navy seal that had spent 28 years in the military. For a chronic low back problem he had an epidural injection in December 2016. In February of 2017 he developed an inguinal or groin abscess that required drainage. This resulted in a spinal abscess where he had the prior epidural. This is not common, but it does happen with no medical fault. It can reflect the underlying suboptimal immune status of the individual.

The infection was MRSA positive. He underwent maximum antibiotic treatment for this and has had multiple problems since that time. Starting in a wheelchair he now has progressed from a walker to a cane. That occurred over two years.

He had progressive left foot drop.

His history also reveals the G.I. issue of frequent, urgent bowel movements 6 to 8 times a day.

All portions of the program are to reboot cells and improve metabolism to what it was years before. This is all about wound healing.

He presented in the middle of the coronavirus pandemic, and I am in NYC. I managed the initial assessment by phone and Skype—pushing 70 and learning to use this technology. The first part of a program is to initiate chemical and hormone optimization.

The patient was started on testosterone which promotes repair and rebuilding with wound healing.

Liposomal NAD (nicotinamide adenine dinucleotide) was initiated to assist with neurologic damage.

An extremely important concept supports the benefit I have seen in MS and many other patients with the use of NAD initially administered using IV infusion. This is not available in conventional hospitals. The use of intravenous NAD was not available for treatment during March through the end of June because of the pandemic. This article basically says when nerve cells are affected by a chronic condition, they dump out all the NAD. This leads to neuropathies but also conditions such as Alzheimer's and Parkinson's may show benefit with NAD intravenous administration. This is where I learn and grow in my current practice.

The best way to restore NAD levels that have dropped is to give initial intravenous infusions. Subsequently, it is difficult to maintain good levels using oral supplements. This can be done but a simpler more reliable method is using liposomal technology as the delivery agent for the NAD to be assimilated optimally. Quicksilver Scientific is a reliable source for good liposomal products. "Liposomes as Advanced Delivery Systems for Nutraceuticals."

Further information about their products can be seen on their website. I do not sell supplements in my office. When I go to an office and see behind the reception desk tons of supplements for sale, I lose confidence in the practitioner. Most New York doctors pad their income by selling supplements. I prefer to give recommendations and directions to patients. I am not a rich doctor, but I am happy to give out reliable recommendations.

Also, when I make a recommendation on treatment, my choice has nothing to do with certain supplements. I look for results. Including the very wealthy, only 5-10% of the population see health from my standpoint. Very few patients would consider a treatment for regeneration if there are no acute symptoms. It is so subtle to get old!!

We also initiated a peptide, BPC 157, by daily subcutaneous injection.

The body has large biological proteins with multiple functions. If a little bit of this protein is taken out this is called a peptide or a short protein. These may have a specific biologic function depending on their origin. The BPC 157 is an agent that overall works well for rehabilitation and tissue recovery. It is of gastrointestinal origin.

Two months after beginning the routine he said his stamina was much better. It had gone from 25% to a 75 to 80% level. He is now exercising six days a week. He also mentioned that he lost 20 pounds and his waist lost 6 inches. His mood is much better. He is sleeping very well. His bowel issues resolved completely. This peptide is of gastrointestinal origin. It frequently aids in common symptoms such as acid reflux, irritable bowel disease, and chronic constipation.

Is this a complicated case? No, this is biohacking.

This is the way to get things to function like they did before using bioidentical substances.

The purpose of this case report is to demonstrate that the body wants to heal itself. Restoring biochemicals leads to improvement in cell function. Improved cell function will help restore immune function.

Peptides are agents to help us function more optimally in certain situations. The use of the peptide is solely for a short period of time.

I adjust the dose of the BPC 157 depending on the patient's presentation during the healing process. A longer course of the BPC 157 could be used or another peptide instituted down the line. I will continue him with BPC 157 for two more months, adding an additional peptide called TB 500. This is also a regenerative peptide that stimulates thymus gland function.

The thymus gland produces T cells which attack viruses.

Stem cells and exosomes assist with wound healing. All portions of the program are to reboot cells and improve metabolism to what it was years before.

HOW I PLAY MY GAME

I spent 29 years in a solo practice doing cardiovascular surgery near Kansas City. I also obtained a doctorate in natural medicine, giving me a wide background and experience with over 45 years in both conventional as well as alternative medical practices. During my surgical career I learned the preoperative evaluation. I operated or helped operate on every part of the body. As a surgeon I was involved with the post op healing process. We had no hospitalists at that time and I rounded on most of my patients twice a day and intensive care unit patients several times a day. There was no dressing team. I saw the wounds daily. Principles learned as a surgeon regarding wound healing are a basic part of my practice including stem cell treatment.

Bio hacking is my game plan. From my surgical background, this is all a matter of wound healing. Agents used in rejuvenation treatment are part of normal biologic substances present, but *depleted*, in our system. As we get older, biochemicals are depleted inside our cells. We need to think about an overhaul, not just an oil change.

My practice is not one where patients come in to get

treated one time and receive a bill. I monitor the patient many times through one or two years as we go through rehabilitation and direct their treatment based on the personal healing response. This is all about wound healing, which is in the larger sense body healing. Stem cells and exosomes assist with regeneration and wound healing.

As the first step, optimization of the patient's chemical and hormone status can be done to promote regeneration and healing. Light (red light to stimulate nitric oxide production) and oxygen are also used as part of stem cell treatment. Interval reappraisal of the patient directs further recommendations for regeneration of tissue. This is where various peptides, like the previously mentioned BPC 157, have come into play as part of the overall picture.

The other common peptide that is used in my rejuvenation program is epitalon. I have one patient who eight years ago had a baseline chronological age of 62 and a biologic age of 56 using telomere measurement. After a health program since that time and one year after epitalon and with a chronologic age of 70 the patient's biologic age was 54 using the same telomere measurement. Biologically younger because of the treatments?? No clinical studies. Just an observation and clinical example. And I have more examples with telomere studies besides myself.

I have minimal gray hair. Body composition is the same as when I was 25 years old. I have been asked if I am Cory's (my son) older brother.

Current epigenetic studies look at methylation of certain portions of the DNA molecule for establishing a biologic age. In my experience telomere measurement is the most accurate way to initially define but also to consistently monitor trending to direct treatment. The downside is it is a little more expensive - $1000. Again, most people, despite valuable information given by the telomere test, feel it will not change their program. As a physician, to develop a program for patients without sufficient hard data may not be successful. Follow up is important.

I promote a rejuvenation program. Think in terms of personal maintenance.

What is the result of this rebooting?

In the future, Part 4 of the book will deal with rebooting and preparing for the second half of the ballgame. Who knows what will happen? Reboot means put on your helmet (and facemask) against the virus as society opens.

My real thought at this point is faithfully wearing masks when outside in crowded areas through the rest of the year unless the government states absolutely no cases of active coronavirus are present. And avoid large and crowded public events.

https://arstechnica.com/science/2020/05/a-look-at-what-covid-patients-are-telling-us-about-the-virus-and-risks/

https://medicine.wustl.edu/news/surprising-culprit-nerve-cell-damage-identified/

46

City Waking Up

28 June 2020

- The New York economy is way down.
- The city is not receiving taxes from visitors.
- Hotels are closed.
- Broadway is closed.
- Subways are about 25% full—and still costing the city a lot of money.
- Life is moving ahead with people beginning to work.
- I have had many patients who have not been able to get any routine medical treatment for many months.
- Because of the fact that New York is an epicenter has curtailed patients from out of country or out of state that normally come in to see me.
- There is little air flight.
- Working over the past three months was really just making some phone calls in follow up while not making much income, trying to pay overhead, and determining what my new game plan will be.

I'm sitting on the balcony watching pedestrians at only about 50% of the normal activity. This has increased slightly the past couple of days because restaurants are now serving outside. After 8 o'clock is very quiet.

There is a concern because currently many patients across the country that are testing positive for coronavirus are in the age range of 20 to 34. This leads to easier spread of the virus. Increased infectivity is still a potential. We're still learning about this and how to handle this pandemic. Answers are not black-and-white even though many people want immediate information, assistance, and no errors.

We are not out of the woods yet. Today (28 June) was reported the largest number of new cases of COVID-19 in the country. This is higher than ever before during this pandemic. The trend is going that direction with no signs of letting up.

I am learning to use Skype for appointments. This is causing a significant technological change in our country.

Telemedicine. It beats having to be in the waiting room with 20 other patients. The only downside is I have to get out of my pajamas.

This scenario has happened to me time and time again when I see a patient for an age management consultation.

A middle-age man (50) comes into my office with a little bit of a paunch and is asked about his medical health. He says his health is pretty good. He exercises and tries to eat right.

As far as medication, he takes something for cholesterol, another for blood pressure, a heart pill, and something for sugar. Oh, a Viagra certainly helps. On his recent annual physical the doctor told him that all his numbers were under control (whatever that means).

I ask you- is this truly healthy? Do you have balance (hormone) for the "human machine" to function optimally? No, he is simply taking prescription pills like so many other middle-aged men. Yet this is accepted by most Americans and for whatever reason seems to be the mindset.

The average lifespan for a man in the country is 76. This patient may not reach that goal because he is going downhill slowly.

His last years may not be quality. All this can be very subtle.

Look at this:

Cholesterol is a precursor used by the body to make sex hormones such as the testosterone. It also is used to make vitamin D. If these are suboptimal (and I am not referring to current conventional medicine reference ranges which may not be optimal and accurate) the cholesterol level rises. If these are optimized the cholesterol level comes down without any medication.

So, the middle-age man goes to the doctor and he passes his physical. However, the doctor says the cholesterol levels are up and hands him another new medicine.

The fact is that elevated cholesterol is really a sign that his metabolism is getting out of whack.

Conventional medicine accepts the fact that the insurance company will pay $3000 a year for cholesterol meds and the patient pays nothing out of pocket. That is the incentive—right or wrong. Their numbers look good, but the metabolism is not optimal. But the system will pay for high cholesterol pills without getting to the root of the problem.

This is so subtle that patients do not identify going slowly downhill.

I have many patients in whom I have discontinued multiple medications after initiating a wellness program. The fact that the insurance company may not cover my exam for testing carries a lot of weight for many patients. They have a low co-pay and do what they are told. Not always smart, but it is the way of the common American.

I try to help patients become more aware so they can make appropriate decisions about their health. It may not be for everyone, but if a person is forward thinking and willing to care for their body then the benefits of longevity can be a key to a continued active life long into the future.

That is what I do.

47

Phase II Here in NYC

1 July 2020

The days are getting shorter. The year is half over.

How about corona? It isn't going away. Most people get over it fairly well, but some are seeing lasting effects. But this is just like any illness; the healthier a person is then the better the body will recover.

How about social settings? No indoor restaurants, hotels, or theater.

We are adjusting so businesses will continue to see revenue. When sidewalks are tight, the city is allowing the curbside driving lanes of the street to be blocked so that nearby restaurants can have outdoor service. Survival.

Restaurants and mom-and-pop businesses are closing. This is a big deal. We haven't seen the government use illness as a means to hinder businesses on this level before.

Most people are wearing masks. Masks are important right now, but can we wear masks for months or years to come? Humans aren't meant to live in masks on this planet.

My son has an interesting perspective in his article he wrote for a publication in the Midwest. He urges people go take safety measures seriously but to look beyond masks to move forward. Your immune system is the best line of defense against future viruses and illnesses.

The statue of Washington got painted red by the rioters. God bless if they ever come across a statue of me!!!

I rode the subway this last week and there were about 10 people per subway car. Physical distancing is still a measure that is usually the easiest to institute. My son says he was social distancing before it was cool. He doesn't like close talkers or touchy people.

NY continues to be strong, but I fear for security if they begin to decrease the police force.

The 7 PM nightly salute has stopped. New York City is into a recovery era and the attitude is to start moving forward. Particularly hurting is tourism with hotels, Broadway plays, theater, and restaurants being closed.

Economically New York City will be recovering for many years. I know I will pay more taxes as they are short a lot of money.

Auto traffic during the week is about 75% to normal. On weekends and holidays the streets are empty—maybe 20%. More and more people are getting out of the city; temporarily or for prolonged periods of time. Some of my wealthy patients have gone to rural Virginia, the northeast New England states, or Colorado and say they are staying away from crowded cities for the foreseeable future.

Medically there are comments about playing around with this virus. This is not the Spanish flu. The concern is that this is a new virus and it mutates regularly. Are we doing the appropriate social protection, and do we learn from this current experience?

This is not the apocalyptic virus, but it helps us get ready for it. Viruses are part of our environment. We will never wipe out all viruses. This is a matter of survival together. There has been information reported indicating that this was a genetic experiment coming from China. Be that as it may. Another severe virus could come from another part of the world. The true key here is personal maintenance.

I emphasize the importance of personal health. Consider personal maintenance and taking your future into your own hands. My system can offer something that the stock market, buying a franchise, or waiting for a vaccine cannot. All I can offer you is the truth about you and how to care for yourself going forward.

You don't have to age grudgingly; your life can be one of grace, enlightenment, and longevity. The first steps are to look within, see how the machine wants to be treated and then do the right thing for yourself. Live right and live long.

Finally, advice from a Massachusetts woman who survived COVID-19, the 1918 flu - and cancer:

After she retired in the late 1980s, she was diagnosed with breast cancer and underwent a lumpectomy and radiation. She beat the disease, but a few years later, doctors diagnosed her with stage 3 colon cancer, from which she also recovered after surgery.

Looking back on her long life, Schappals - who struggles with periodic memory lapses but is otherwise very sharp - said she is satisfied and happy. She advises young people to be positive and honest with themselves. And she offers this insight: "Most people are innately good and sympathetic," she said. "They want to do the right thing, but it's easy to be sidetracked by selfishness and emotion."

"The more things change, the more they remain the same," Schappals said. *"I believe that now."*

Is there anything else she wants to add?

"Yeah," she told her daughter. "When can we go for a car ride?"

https://www.stamfordadvocate.com/lifestyle/article/Advice-from-a-woman-who-survived-covid-19-the-15454667.php

http://www.emporiagazette.com/free/article_deee8d86-bf90-11ea-85b4-23f64bcf3697.html

https://www.express.co.uk/news/world/1317588/China-coronavirus-cover-up-scientist-military-lab-wet-market-where-did-coronavirus-start

III

Part Three

Now we move forward in the world, learning how to do so together.

48

How Long Until the Medicine Takes?

I am in Manhattan and this is 6 PM Sunday, **July 12**. I am on my fourth-floor balcony making phone calls and doing paperwork. A young guy in his late 20s came walking by on the sidewalk carrying a surfboard. He must have been at Coney Island or a New Jersey beach. New Jersey people do not like New York people coming down and invading their state right now. Incidence of coronavirus is way down here in NYC, but still up some in New Jersey. Cuomo declares 14-day quarantine for out of state people coming to NYC. Recovery will be slow.

Despite hot weather, Florida rates are up. So is California. They are beginning to restrict restaurants, bars, and movie theaters. Social distancing is very important. And it is not forever. Only with an epidemic.

Parts 1 and 2 in this series contain a journal, personal adventures, observations, and health aspects during the onset of the COVID-19 pandemic from the epicenter in New York City.

271

We are still learning. Many people expect instant information, immediate assistance, and no errors. This does not exist in the real world with the COVID-19 pandemic.

In Part 3 we begin to approach some health and medical information that:

1. *Uses lay terminology so the scientific information is understood.*
2. *Enables you to be more informed about this particular pandemic.*
3. *Allows you to become aware of health methods not promoted by conventional medicine.*

In this portion of the book aspects of biohacking to reboot cells to work more optimally will be presented. There are no drugs involved. This involves restoring biologic agents that have depleted with time. This is very subtle. Society accepts "you are just getting older." After time there is significant deterioration of cell function that leads to the development of chronic and degenerative conditions. This process can be reversed.

https://www.linkedin.com/pulse/what-does-mean-reboot-joseph-edward-bosiljevac-jr-md-phd-facs/

https://www.linkedin.com/pulse/personal-maintenance-reversibility-bosiljevac-jr-md-phd-facs/?trackingId=1UPb%2F%2BUy nansYf3R2REz2A%3D%3D

49

Where are we Now? What is the Game Plan? OK.

We have never established a national program using extensive testing to delineate the epidemiology of a viral infection. There are medical aspects to be gained from scientific information accumulated with the current COVID-19. This is information that can be used in the future with other epidemics. We live in a world that has viruses and viruses will never be eliminated. This is the importance of personal maintenance. We need to learn to survive.

As far as the medical aspects of this particular virus, I will not get into the argument whether this is an engineered virus developed to establish an epidemic outside of China for financial and political reasons. This could happen from many other sources in the world.

There are thoughts that this may not be like other viruses. My contention as a scientist is to believe this will act biologically as we know so far from the knowledge of past and current viral studies.

So where do we stand?

- First of all, we are in **recovery**. Maybe. Overall incidence is increasing.
- Incidence is down significantly in New York, but now increasing in Florida, Texas, and Arizona.
- Miami is now the new epicenter (July 14).

There have been precautions to control high risk populations, so the death rate is less than it is in New York City. Another bigger outbreak could occur around October.

Everyone wants immunity. **Resistance**.

Everyone worries about antibody positivity which means you are protected from the infection and not carrying the virus to give to anyone else.

Other than widespread disease to develop immunity, how do we handle this?

My thoughts:

1. You get the infection and develop protective antibodies.
2. Cross antibody protection from other viruses may protect from this and potentially other future viruses. The Corona and the bird flu virus are not the same virus, but cross-reactivity could play a part to produce antibodies effective with COVID-19 or other viruses.
3. Vaccination may soon be available and here is where we can begin to establish herd immunity.

Antibody function has variables that rely on the underlying health of the individual (if a patient is healthy, they may be extremely resistant and not even develop an infection or antibodies). It also depends on the amount of exposure to the virus as far as infectivity. If the immune ability of the patient is low antibodies may not form even after active infection. Also, there may be some difference between individuals. This is what I have seen taking care of my patient population.

Look at the experience in Hong Kong without a lockdown. This was also seen in Vietnam, South Korea, and Japan.

They follow government direction:

1. Avoid enclosed spaces with poor ventilation.
2. Avoid crowded places with many people.
3. Avoid close contact settings such as face-to-face conversations without a mask.
4. The government may also declare a medical emergency where nursing homes and high-risk patients are protected.

Officials also tried to track down and quarantine all the people who any COVID-19 patients had seen two days before becoming sick. Anyone arriving from mainland China or another infected country were also required to stay in a 14-day quarantine at home or at designated facility before entering. Social distancing, *flexible work schedules, and school closures were also used to help stop the spread.*

"If these measures and population responses can be sustained, while avoiding fatigue among the general population, they could substantially lessen *the impact of a local COVID-19 epidemic,"* Cowling added.*

This is the Japanese experience. They have had a mysteriously low virus death rate. There are many theories but it really boils down to how they treat their bodies and what they ingest.

Heavy breathing in close proximity is the biggest factor in promoting the spread of the virus. Enclosed spaces with poor ventilation are areas of highest risk. This is the big risk with schools.

Look at the Swedish experience with no lockdown. Somewhat successful. We are still learning as a society how to handle this.

Open markets increase exposure. Masks and social distancing are essential to minimize exposure. Other disinfecting items and ultraviolet lights may also be useful.

Masks are easily accepted in Asia from their epidemic experience starting with the Spanish flu in 1918. In Asian countries if the government says wear a mask it is either that, a big fine, or jail.

Americans have never seen this kind of directive on a national basis. There are complaints about interference with personal rights. We are talking about individual rights sometimes restricted because of social benefit. During an epidemic wearing a mask is a respect item. At other times if people have a cough or cold a mask should be expected. Protect high risk patients and those in nursing homes. And back off large public events for the present time. Communities with surges in COVID-19 cases should take three steps to slow the transmission of the virus according to Admiral Brett Giroir, MD, HHS assistant secretary Thursday:

1. Close bars and limit seating in restaurants.
2. Have people avoid crowds.
3. Get at least 90% of people to wear masks when out in public.

School openings are a big deal right now. Different routines have been performed in other countries. The main thing is distancing. Perhaps the class could go online half day and in the classroom half day. Class size should be limited to about 15 maximum. Testing can be performed on students to try to limit exposure. It is important to promote fresh air. Maybe the student should start with online to start the year and proceed depending on the status of the epidemic.

Trained dogs can smell coronavirus. This may be useful when disinfecting a large facility following a crowded event.

Medical conditions like obesity can increase risk of infection and complications. Many Americans are not functioning optimally with their metabolism. They expect if they get sick medicine will help them.

Current medical knowledge does not provide a specific protocol to follow during an epidemic. There are no straightforward medical treatments to recover from this infection. We are learning as we go. Asians have learned to do this.

We also need to learn to survive. The struggle here is economics and lifestyle recovery such as opening schools and restaurants. Air travel also needs to increase. We really need to be looking at opening up society with appropriate social measures. Many people do not understand that we are still learning.

In Asian countries it may not be COVID-19 but a similar virus that occurred in the past which has left a long-standing immunity with various generations. SARS virus (like corona) has circulated in this region before. This may also explain a lower death rate because of prior immunity. We are learning. This is a corona virus, which is different than the bird flu.

How significant is that? We keep being thrown curveballs - which just means we are still learning.

We are learning about infectivity. The SARS virus was infective to only about 20% of the population. We really do not have any hard or fast evidence regarding testing with another prior epidemic. If COVID-19 is more contagious than SARS it may require 80% of the population to have antibodies to develop herd immunity. In this fashion we are learning as a nation how to handle this pandemic. The best way right now as a nation is a vaccination program.

The development of a vaccine for coronavirus is at a good point with the AstraZeneca research. Stage I apparently had 145 patients. Stage II the vaccine was administered to 30,000 patients. Results showed higher levels of antibodies in these people than those that were naturally infected. The next is Stage III to see how long the antibody lasts and also if there are any significant side effects with more time.

According to the FDA the vaccine will be available for the public early 2021.

I heard an interview on Hannity. He was talking with Dr. Oz. When Oz was asked "From what you know about the research on the AstraZeneca vaccine, would you take it now?" He answered with a resounding yes.

Dr. Oz may be better than a clinical study. It shows the line of thinking from a medical scientist.

The government has a lot of barriers trying to control the right balance and avoid damage. Perhaps some of those barriers need to be eased to help the economic aspects of the pandemic.

An early vaccination program may be our victory with coronavirus.

One thing to consider is accuracy of the testing. In one year, we will know more. This is the first American epidemic that is trying new scientific means for extensive testing. The accuracy and how this directs what can be done at the onset of another epidemic are to be learned. Despite testing recommended by WHO - extensive testing has never been done. We do not have that information available to direct how best socially to control an epidemic.

Remember what was done without a lockdown in Hong Kong and other Asian countries. We do not have to prove things with a strict clinical trial to decide whether you need to wear a mask or not. Some things are common sense and respect items. Hopefully a more specific study of the epidemiology of this virus will add further helpful medical information. Opening of bars, restaurants, and schools are the major social aspects pending at this time.

There will be continued exposure to zoonotic viruses. This refers to the ability of the virus to transfer from another animal to human. The bird flu virus is an example. So is the pig virus. Coronavirus happens to be transmitted frequently by bats.

Plan ahead. This is not the apocalyptic virus. If this coronavirus was an engineered virus then something even more virulent could present itself down the line. We need to protect our future with increased personal hygiene and health.

A point I would like to make is that as we start Part 3 (and who knows how many parts there will be) I will try to share my background and experience in health to direct patients with their own personal health. Social management of an epidemic is important but the health aspects for yourself should also be a priority. My goal is to provide medical information to patients at the lay level so it is understood. Then the patient will make appropriate health decisions for themselves.

In this portion of the book, aspects of biohacking to reboot cells to work more optimally will be presented. There are no drugs involved. This involves restoring biologic agents that have depleted with time. This is very subtle. Society accepts "you are just getting older." After time there is significant deterioration of cell function that leads to the development of chronic and degenerative conditions. This process many times can be reversed.

Cells have suboptimal function because biological agents in the cell have become depleted. The rejuvenation program is something that restores these agents.

This is called **rebooting** cells.

A contention I make is this:

A healthy 50-year-old can do a rejuvenation program to restore biologic agents depleted in their cells (reboot cells). If the cells work more optimally the improved metabolic function may be that of a 35-year-old. Chronologic age continues to go up. A true age management program pushes biologic age down. The level of metabolic function improves. Biohacking. Rebooting. Regeneration. Rejuvenation.

The downturn with aging can be very subtle and it is important to identify essentials to provide a good age management program. This includes extensive bloodwork. This process is diagnostic to provide data points that can be used to assess recovery. We are talking about subtle symptoms.

As part of an age management practice I find that body parts wear out. 12 years ago, I started with retired NFL and NBA players and began learning about stem cell injections in joints. Results over the years have been very good. In 80% of my patients no other treatment including surgery was ever necessary.

With my continued involvement with military special forces groups, I have used intravenous infusions and other methods to deliver stem cells given for systemic conditions. Some of these were lung problems, heart and liver problems, and traumatic brain injury with highly satisfactory results and no harm.

I have expanded what I learned to treat many patients who have an autoimmune or other chronic neurodegenerative condition. As they go through a rejuvenation program the result may be the resolution of some of the symptoms.

I had an elderly woman with MS who had painful neuropathy in both legs requiring 6-8 opioid pain pills daily. During the first part of the rejuvenation program the administration of intravenous NAD immediately relieved the painful neuropathy. That was only temporary and long-term resolution was obtained after the stem cell treatment. One month after stem cells she required no pain pills.

Before the rejuvenation program this patient was seeing 10 different specialists and the entire weekly schedule was filled going to different exams and treatments. Besides the resolution of the painful neuropathy she eliminated a good portion of her other symptoms and now has a more direct, simple program with only three doctors. She is in her mid-80s, lives with her husband in her private home and drives a car. She was not able to drive prior to her treatment—she never could parallel park. Ha. Ha. She is driving now. And she continues to learn. She tells her husband that health wise she cannot do the dishes!

Symptomatically, all patients feel much improved from what they were experiencing before a rejuvenation treatment. You are getting the body to work better. This is more effective than supplements. This is an overhaul and not an oil change.

This is so basic to understand. Most people don't get it. They spend money to keep their apartment or home in good shape, maintain an automobile, motorhome, motorcycle, buy expensive workout equipment, and they do maintenance on other items in their life. But to do a <u>personal</u> maintenance program?

A rejuvenation program is simply regeneration. Wound healing. The body works better.

Rebooting is one of the next chapters in this part of the book, and we will build on that with topics that include NAD, exosomes, peptides, diet, exercise, and even stem cells.

Where does the word **okay** come from? I'm a Midwesterner from Kansas/Nebraska. This is a Cherokee word (okey) that means "all is good." **BIOHACKING.** *Rebooting. Regeneration. Rejuvenation. OK.*

https://www.newsweek.com/sweden-which-never-had-lockdown-sees-covid-19-cases-plummet-rest-europe-suffers-spike-1521626

50

Epicenter NYC

10 July 2020

We are here:

Early recovery. Not only personal health, but economics and that of lifestyle and society. The other goal is resistance.

It is possible COVID-19 is a newly engineered virus developed by the Chinese. The bird flu and corona are different viruses. We have not really studied the epidemiology of this particular virus. We are still learning. Many people expect immediate information, assistance, and no errors. We are not there yet.

Are we prepared for the true apocalyptic virus? Coronavirus is not this.

The incidence of coronavirus and the death rate in New York have markedly diminished. However, the rest of the country is seeing an increase of cases and death rate. Maybe we are slightly ahead in the ballgame here in the city, but this pandemic is not over.

I emphasize personal health is essential for resistance and recovery.

Here are some of my present thoughts which includes testing of patients in my practice and what has been found with other testing done here in New York City. Keep in mind that in the real world not everything is black and white clear. We are dealing with a situation where there are multiple variables.

1. There are 1% of people that have positive antibodies to the virus. Half of these people never remember any known illness.

2. Other states show lower mortality than New York perhaps by keeping nursing homes and elderly disabled patients isolated.

3. The pattern I see is that many people are asymptomatic but can be carriers if they have antibodies from prior other virus infections like the bird flu protecting them from an infection like COVID-19. They do not form specific antibodies to COVID-19 and they do not develop an active infection but maintain the carrier state. They are medically very healthy.

4. COVID-19 appears to be reasonably infective so up to 70 or 80 percent of the population may need to develop antibodies to provide herd immunity for overall society. Hopefully, this can be done with vaccination instead of actively infected patients.

5. Antibodies develop in most patients after an active and also an inactive or asymptomatic illness.

6. NY City is into a recovery era. Particularly hurting is tourism with hotels, Broadway plays, theater, and

restaurants closed. 60 million annual tourists are missing.

7. My professional practice is struggling. Many patients are gone and not coming back to NYC for a long time. No income since March.

8. It is expensive to survive on an island. I have not left Manhattan since December 2019. My rents have not changed.

9. There has been some rioting and destruction here in NYC and elsewhere. The Columbus statue was painted red and statues elsewhere have been pulled down.

10. Maybe lines are now short to get to the top of the Empire State Building.

I had a patient in the office recently who lives in Brooklyn. He had not gone into Manhattan for three months and began to drive to his office in midtown three days a week about a month ago. As I reviewed his experience with the coronavirus it was as follows:

1. He had a sister become ill and expire during the pandemic.

2. He has a construction business and everything was upside down. He says this is beginning to stabilize.

3. Traffic into Manhattan is not too bad. This week he was able to drive 60 miles an hour going into Manhattan. But traffic is getting heavier each week.

4. His office is in midtown and he feels the city appears more sleazy. It has lost its charm and there are too many vagrants and homeless around with no open businesses.

Both street and pedestrian traffic is really down.

Masks are important as well as social distancing while the virus is active is important. There are no magic bullets. **Personal health.** I say this a lot. **I feel very few patients truly understand what I say about rebooting and regeneration. Biohacking. Rejuvenation.**

https://www.linkedin.com/pulse/personal-maintenance-reversibility-bosiljevac-jr-md-phd-facs/?trackingId=1UPb%2F%2BUy nansYf3R2REz2A%3D%3D

https://www.linkedin.com/pulse/apocalyptic-virus-joseph-edward-bosiljevac-jr-md-phd-facs/?trackingId=x930VCZ4Qq27T4nC

51

Dr. Reboot and Biohacking

I have been through various stages in my life. The first was growing up and finishing college. The second portion was going through medical school and surgical training. At the age of 30 I began my clinical practice, the big third stage of my life.

Halfway through my practice of cardiovascular surgery, I became frustrated because patients presented for surgery and they were on 20 different medications, had tried various alternative methods that improved their condition, but overall were not medically healthy. At that point I obtained a doctorate in natural medicine over a period of about three years while I had a full-time solo surgical practice. For many years I combined conventional medicine with alternative methods from natural medicine such as prolozone injections of joints.

After 29 years of solo practice near Kansas City, I had an offer to move to New York City and open an age management office. I was single. My children were grown. This trip to New York City has been the next adventure in my life the past 12 years.

The most recent episode is the pandemic with the Corona virus. This has provided many challenges medically and socially. I lived in the epicenter the past 4 months. The epicenter is now Miami. We are learning about the progression and evolution of the disease. Our world is filled with viruses. These viruses will never be eliminated completely. Although the coronavirus has been a little threatening with its presentation, this is not the apocalyptic virus.

The information I give to you is from my background and experience and clinical practice with thousands of patients. There is a difference in opinion sometimes from clinical experimental scientists and those that actually do face-to-face patient care.

In conventional medicine and surgical training, I learned to do the preoperative evaluation and the judgment call whether a surgical procedure was necessary. I learned to do surgery. During my training and career, I have operated or helped operate on every part of the human body. When I was in training there were no hospitalists. I made twice daily rounds on all my surgical patients. I became very familiar with the principles of wound healing.

The use of stem cells presents an opportunity with regeneration of tissue and rejuvenation.

When I began doing stem cell therapy, I noticed results improved dramatically when I followed certain wound care healing principles. It is not a matter of just giving someone a shot and you're done with it. No. This is regeneration and wound healing and further treatment is dictated by the healing course of the patient.

I will present clinical stories noted during my career.

These are observations which helped me learn more. As a clinical scientist, when I see consistent results with several patients it attracts my attention and may affect my judgment.

There may be no formal studies on some of the things I present. I try to use lay terms so that the patient can decide whether this information is worthwhile or not for their health.

Biohacking is not complex. Here is a simple understanding about cells that will help to understand the rebooting process. Biochemicals inside the cell deplete with age. The cell function begins to degrade and eventually degenerative conditions and even can evolve. These substances can be rebooted. This is a true overhaul and not an oil change.

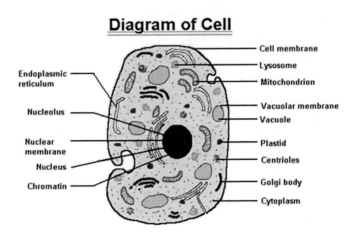

Diagram of Cell

Cell membrane
Lysosome
Endoplasmic reticulum
Mitochondrion
Nucleolus
Vacuolar membrane
Vacuole
Nuclear membrane
Plastid
Nucleus
Centrioles
Chromatin
Golgi body
Cytoplasm

The biologic unit that provides function for our body is a cell. Most cells contain a nucleus. The nucleus contains the DNA which is the genetic material. Think of the DNA strand as a shoestring. The little plastic aglets on each end of the shoestring represent telomeres. When the cell divides the DNA replicates and the telomeres (aglets) shorten. After time the telomeres are short enough that the DNA cannot replicate any further. The bottom line here is that if you prevent telomeres from shortening or actually increase the length of the telomere then you have become biologically younger.

Mitochondria are the energy machines in the cell. Energy production requires CoQ10, which can deplete with age. This can be taken as a supplement. The other important item here is NAD (nicotinamide adenine dinucleotide).

NAD is a coenzyme that helps scoot along the process of energy production in the cell known as the Krebs cycle. If normal energy is produced there is good optimal function. If energy levels begin to go down, then very subtly this can lead to a long-standing degenerative or chronic condition or even cancer. NAD levels get low as we get older. Patients with chronic neurodegenerative conditions have nerve cells that have dumped out the NAD. These patients develop neuropathies. I have seen neuropathies disappear completely with intravenous infusion of NAD. In this condition you're just filling up the gas tank and the improvement is only temporary. A long-standing result may include stem cell treatment. By age 50, including those who consider themselves in great shape, most have had a significant decrease in their NAD levels since childhood.

Figure 6.11A An overview of the Krebs cycle

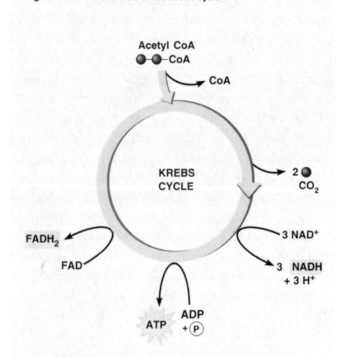

The cell membrane is very important. You can see on the diagram of the cell some indentations in the outer cell membrane.

Inside the cell are little pockets that contain biologic proteins. These are called endosomes or lysosomes. Sometimes an endosome will go through the cell membrane to float free in the open circulation and can go to any part of the body. At this time it is called an exosome. Exosomes serve as growth factors for wound healing and regeneration.

The inside of the cell is made up of water which also contains trace minerals and other things such as toxic heavy metals. Biologic proteins and chemicals are present. Viruses and bacteria can invade the cell if they get through the outer cell membrane. Health aspects related to this will be covered down the line. Most Americans are actually dehydrated inside the cell. This occurs despite significant water consumed every day. Processed water is not effective to move inside the cell. Lack of trace minerals can also affect the movement of water into and out of the cell.

Liposomes are fatty molecules that make up the normal cell membrane. With aging these liposomes are replaced by bad fats and the cell membrane becomes more rigid. This results in the membrane being non-pliable and can affect muscle and tendon strength and flexibility. As we get older it is easier to develop injuries for this reason.

Liposomal encapsulation is available as a delivery agent. There are some medications that cannot be absorbed by mouth. To put a chemical such as glutathione or EDTA with liposomes and apply an ultrasound will create little spheres of the liposomes which surround the particular substance. Since the liposomes can pass easily through the cell membrane, they deliver these agents directly into the cell.

So, in this case the liposomes serve as a delivery agent and then they can be used by the cell to restore the cell membrane.

A source I trust is *Quicksilver Scientific*. A clear liposomal solution contains smaller liposomes that are absorbed better. Liposomal NAD is available for supplementation after initial intravenous dosing of the NAD.

Of the large biologic proteins, small pieces can be removed. Then you have a short protein called a **peptide**. Since the large biologic proteins have multiple functions, a peptide can be processed for a specific biologic activity in the body. This can include regeneration and repair, stimulation of the thymus gland function for immune system benefit, affect cell growth in skin and hair, improve insulin resistance, and lengthen telomeres (which makes you biologically younger).

Hormones are an important aspect for healing. Hormones are biologic chemicals that have local as well as systemic effects. The body is a hormone orchestra which has various sections such as the thyroid, adrenal gland, pituitary gland, and sex hormones. Many of these hormones promote healing. If there are multiple deficiencies in the hormone sections and one is improved than other sections may also 'play better' without any specific treatment. This is part of the overall wound healing plan that promotes the orchestra to sound better and better.

AGE MANAGEMENT – WOUND HEALING

With an age management practice, I found that patients have body parts that wear out. My experience with stem cells started with joint and soft tissue injections and includes treating retired NFL and NBA players as well as men from military special forces. I have followed the course of stem cell treatments extracting fat or bone marrow as the stem cell source, PRP, and placental stem cell products. The last four years I have limited my practice to the use of umbilical cord stem cells. Part of the experience I have gained over the last 12 years is that after age 40 I may not want your own stem cells.

I am currently certified in stem cell therapies. This is where the concept of wound healing has been essential for beneficial results. I follow the principle of **First Do No Harm.**

Review this history of a patient who suffered a COVID-19 infection four months ago but continues with recurrent symptoms. Be aware that using a rejuvenation program approach on autoimmune patients is frequently very helpful. Rebooting cells to function optimally. This patient is suffering from an autoimmune condition, which just means this infection threw her immune system out of whack. Rebooting cells can improve and reverse autoimmune conditions.

I do not have a recipe and follow principles of wound healing learned as a surgeon. I thoroughly evaluate the patient using the human machine concept. Chemical and hormone balance is restored. The condition to be treated is evaluated to determine how the stem cells will be administered. An overall treatment program is developed using adjunctive services to promote healing and recovery.

Light therapy, oxygen, establishing chemical and hormone balance, and certain biologic substances such as NAD are essential adjuvants of the healing process. I rarely see these components provided in U.S. practice. The use of these modalities require certification.

BIOHACKING. *Rebooting. Regeneration. Rejuvenation.*

Information learned from my stem cell experience and wound healing principles has also been beneficial in confronting coronavirus. Now we will cover in more detail the process of bio hacking.

After reading this chapter, if a rejuvenation program would cost $15,000, would you be willing to do that? That kind of money may be spent on things for the house or a motorcycle. Most will not invest this for themselves even though additional quality time can be added to your life. What is that worth? Hopefully as specific details of rebooting and rejuvenation are presented in subsequent chapters, this may lead some people to seriously consider this option which truly is age-management.

https://www.linkedin.com/pulse/apocalyptic-virus-joseph-edward-bosiljevac-jr-md-phd-facs/?trackingId=x930VCZ4Qq27T4

https://www.linkedin.com/pulse/what-does-mean-reboot-joseph-edward-bosiljevac-jr-md-phd-facs/

https://www.linkedin.com/pulse/personal-maintenance-reversibility-bosiljevac-jr-md-phd-facs/?trackingId=1UPb%2F%2Bt nansYf3R2REz2A%3D%3D

https://blogs.webmd.com/my-experience/20200716/i-got-covid19-4-months-ago-i-still-live-with-symptoms?ecd=wnl_spr_0 spr-071620_nsl-LeadModule_title&mb=lGVdiurmHBMQOzQukn

52

Back to School

Mid July

- 17 July was noted to have the highest daily incidence in the overall country of the coronavirus.
- Sitting on my balcony I spot a Jeep that drives by with large letters: **DAD PROUD of the GRAD.**
- This same day walking home from the office (July 17) I walked by a car that was decorated right and left and upside down and in between for a married couple. There was so much going on with that car because they spent the flower money for the church on the car.
- The American Academy of Pediatrics stated that the biggest goal is to get kids back in school and have established some criteria.
- No nation has tried to send children back to school with the virus raging at levels like they are in the United States.
- The WHO has concluded that the virus spread is airborne. Closed spaces with poor ventilation are bad.

- People think that online is easy. Many children do not have computers or if they have computers loaned from the school, they may not have Internet available at home. They need school and discipline.
- There have been no strict scientific studies but case reports from other countries are available. There will be a lot of subclinical infection. We cannot eliminate that. The need is to minimize out of school spread.
- Elementary schools are safer than high schools. I think there's too much kissing in the latter. Physical distancing and masks are essential.
- There are a lot of people working on this. We are still learning. No one knows all the facts and it is difficult to predict the future.
- Keep in mind many people believe that we can automatically find instant information that is absolutely correct. However, we are learning.
- We are still learning medically as well how socially to handle this pandemic.

There is no specific national protocol for opening schools in the pandemic with the coronavirus. I emphasize that we are still learning. We are learning medical aspects about the virus. We are learning as a country the social aspects and lifestyle changes that go along with a viral pandemic.

There are some recent international studies demonstrating how this has been attempted in other countries. There have not been rigorous scientific studies on the potential for school-based spread with COVID-19. These countries indicate a low risk of transmission but without formal testing.

In Ireland, restrictions on class size is the main requirement. There does not appear to be a lot of documented transmission of the virus in this study, but there was no formal testing, and this was back in March.

In Norway and Denmark they opened elementary schools with limited testing. Students were not required to wear a mask and were in smaller classes. Bathroom breaks allowed only a few students at a time to use the facility. Neither country has seen a significant increase in cases.

In Israel the school is closed if there is an outbreak in that facility.

In France 2 high school teachers became ill with COVID-19 in early February and the school closed. On closing they found antibodies in 38% of the students, 43% of the teachers, and 59% of other school workers. Obviously, this shows that the virus circulates without significant infection.

In Germany no mask is required if the student tests negative for the virus. The goal is to restrict mask usage by younger children.

So, after reviewing these recommendations our CDC has no hard and fast rules on how to handle school openings. It is not easy just to do things 'on line.'

Some students may not have computers. Even if provided by school, some homes do not have Internet. The students learn not only by computer but also intraclass activity. And there are the interactions with other students. The social aspect of learning.

Obviously, the first obstacle to overcome is distancing. Although this still makes it difficult for working parents to manage, the student begins doing online first to see what the status of COVID-19 in September. Then classes could be online half a day and in class half a day trying to limit class size to 10 - 15 students. Testing is limited at this time. It is important to promote fresh air and keep the windows open.

So, there will be a transition most likely rather than hard and fast rules that don't change. The half a day distancing to some degree is an aspect that cuts down on contact but may not help working parents. Control over bathrooms should be provided. Ultraviolet lights can be used in the classroom continuously at night to disinfect.

This also gives us a time to be able to teach our children the respect aspect such as wearing a mask and handwashing.

With this pandemic we are learning not only in the medical sense but also social living and personal hygiene.

What I look at is:

1. Hybrid days which may or may not work well with families that have two working parents.
2. Kids that are sick or with a runny nose should stay at home.
3. Parents need to stay away from entering the school.
4. Obviously distancing and wearing a mask are essential.
5. Limiting the number of people in the bathroom at one time and having more effective ventilation.
6. Having more testing available. The school nurse could help isolate patients that are asymptomatic carriers.
7. Hallways can be directed one way. This is rather simple but could be helpful when I think in terms of the congestion in the halls of the school.
8. This is an opportunity for children to learn better social and personal hygiene.

I come out with another comment. Nose spray. Look at the evidence from the British group of healthcare workers that used iodine to kill the coronavirus that was on the surface in the nose or the throat.

So, before the kid goes to school and when he comes home at night he gets a spray in each nose and a spray in his mouth. This is effective, convenient, and inexpensive. You will never see this used to any degree. A patented product is necessary to make a profit. I do not do my work to make money. This is a very simple measure just like using ultraviolet rays at night in the workplace or school to kill virus.

The dental profession is aware of this including effective-ness against many coronavirus.

https://www.nature.com/articles/s41415-020-1589-4

https://www.linkedin.com/pulse/16-april-i-came-across-release-from-british-group-joseph-edward/?trackingId=gVLHzmpEw

https://www.webmd.com/lung/news/20200710/as-cases-surge-no-clear-answers-on-school-reopening?ecd=wnl_spr_071120&spr-071120_nsl-LeadModule_title&mb=lGVdiurmHB-MQOzQukn1aapAyWFWqf9PLEH%2foKnlpKv4%3d

https://www.hippocraticpost.com/covid-19-update/iodine-nasal-spray-and-mouthwash-may-protect-healthworkers/

https://clinicaltrials.gov/ct2/show/NCT04364802

53

Cholesterol Medication and Corona Make This a 'Common Cold'?

I have previously presented medical items as far as acute treatment of COVID-19. Let me review some of these as we come across information that an anti-cholesterol drug could be a helpful agent to fight the current coronavirus.

Monolaurin is more of a preventive agent. However, it has a good antiviral effect and can shorten illness if the dosage is increased above maintenance when symptoms occur.

Dexamethasone, which is a very powerful cortisone type medication, has been helpful in some patients. This is also useful in many cases of severe infection and stress.

Hydroxychloroquine has also been evaluated. The press took off on this, in fact, when President Trump took this for two weeks. I happen to know one of the President's former physicians in New York City. During that time, he said that his office was being overwhelmed with phone calls from news agencies to find out if he was the one that had prescribed the medication.

Ozone has been found helpful to improve the oxygen

status in patients. However, ozone is also antimicrobial and antiviral.

Case presentations are helpful, and I remember morbidity and mortality conferences regularly held during my surgical training. Learn from experience. This case presentation shows thinking outside the box of conventional medicine. It introduces the concept of using glutathione.

Coronavirus can cause serious lung problems. The case summary tells about a medical student who took the advice of Dr. David Horowitz, a Lyme disease specialist. He recommended 2000 mg of glutathione. Glutathione leads to break down of mucus in the lungs, so it is not clumped together.

I will not get into scientific details about glutathione - there is other literature out there. Glutathione promotes cellular health. It inhibits virus. The antiviral quality is that rebooting cells leads to improved cell function. It can affect the natural killer cell activity of T cells, so it boosts the immune system.

It is not well absorbed when taken by mouth. In this particular case she responded to oral medication. If you look at the label the medication is in 50 mg capsules. So, she took well above the recommended dose with the 2000 mg!

No.

My final comment - Dr. Horowitz, what a brilliant judgment call demonstrating your experience and ability to think outside the box.

IV infusion is best, and I usually give 1000 milligrams at a time. This could be given 2 to 3 times a day in severely ill patients.

Liposomal glutathione would also be effectively absorbed.

A source I trust is *Quicksilver Scientific*. A clear liposomal solution contains smaller liposomes that are absorbed better. Sublingual is convenient and can be very effective.

Of the items mentioned to this point, the other thing to consider is personal health. Many people think if they get sick that current medical treatment will make them well. I emphasize again that the human machine needs to be ready to heal.

This is where I get into rebooting cells. This is more important than any particular medication that has been demonstrated to this point with coronavirus.

There have been several European studies demonstrating smokers have a lower incidence of corona infection.

French researchers to give nicotine patches to coronavirus patients and frontline workers after lower rates of infection were found among smokers. There was a study that demonstrated CBD had an effect by blocking the gateway for the virus to enter the lining of the nose or the throat.

This appears to be related to angiotensin converting enzyme 2 receptors (ACE). These can be blocked by CBD which helps produce an anti-inflammatory effect.

ACE receptors are very common as the entryway for some heart and blood pressure medication. This expands to CBD because it has been shown that these ACE receptors are the landing point and entry site for the coronavirus.

What does this mean? This is not a magic cure to defeat coronavirus but simply demonstrates the mechanism of biologic activity, particularly things that influence the ACE 2 receptor. Many of the medications that affect these receptors are administered for high blood pressure and heart and blood vessel problems. These may affect receptor sites and could influence the infection rate, but this has not been noted to be a major problem. Patients are directed to continue their medications for chronic conditions and not change any during the pandemic.

Two doctors from New York Mount Sinai Medical Center have discovered information regarding a cholesterol-lowering drug fenofibrate (Tricor) to treat COVID-19 patients.

Trying to understand the process of lung damage that occurred with the SARS CoV-2 infection in the past, they found that the virus prevents the routine burning of carbohydrates. Subsequently, there would be fat accumulation inside the lung cells enabling the virus to reproduce. So their line of thinking is to use a cholesterol lowering drug to decrease fat accumulation inside the patient's lungs.

Again, as I tell you this, keep in mind that we are talking about altering metabolism in cells. I presented information in the previous chapter on the Krebs cycle as far as an energy production mechanism for each cell. If the energy level goes down there may be only some very subtle changes, nothing that causes you to go to the emergency room. But the cells are not working optimum. Regardless of whatever kind of microorganism attempts to attack us in the future, we need to have the home fortress stable. Personal health. Rebooting cells which sometimes cannot be done very well by oral supplements.

A five-day treatment with this cholesterol medication resulted in absence of virus in every patient treated.

Is this effective? This is not a clinical study, but it shows progressive medical thinking. A five-day treatment with fenofibrate may be very effective to reduce the second wave. They comment that that would make the second wave more of a common cold.

I am going to take this a step further.

A 55-year-old man goes through his annual checkup with the doctor who says "Everything looks good. However, you need to lose a little bit of weight and here is a prescription for a cholesterol medication based on you blood tests."

Cholesterol is a useful chemical that is used as a precursor to form vitamin D and also sex hormones. Most Americans have low vitamin D levels. At age 55 this guy is probably having some drop in his testosterone from his optimal physiologic level - the level of his hormone where he runs an optimal human machine.

If the cholesterol is elevated, then treatment of suboptimal testosterone and vitamin D levels will bring the cholesterol down without any medication! I see this all the time. And what is difficult is accepting reference ranges in conventional medicine as optimal. Patients are told "Oh, you are in the normal range. You don't need testosterone." If a 55-year-old man has a testosterone level that is 10 or 15% of the level when he was 35 years old, then his system is running sub optimally. Cholesterol levels go up. Sugar metabolism gets worse and adult onset diabetes comes on.

Two courses occur here. Take medication and accept health decline 'that comes with aging.' Reboot your system to work normal and take no medication. This stuff works!

Cholesterol drugs have made a lot of money in our medical

system. The question is whether it is truly effective or not. It makes certain numbers on annual bloodwork look better, but survival?

So, my thought is this:

A five- or 10-day treatment of the drug fenofibrate at the onset of a viral illness like corona could be a winner. Although I think most cholesterol medication is given to patients who have suboptimal hormone and vitamin D levels, this clinical practice of prescribing cholesterol medication to patients will probably be continued. However, if there was a cut back in the use of cholesterol medication as in the patient above, then the possible use for treating coronavirus and other viruses will provide a marketplace.

So where are we overall?

I also need to push rebooting cells and personal maintenance.

https://www.linkedin.com/pulse/what-does-mean-reboot-joseph-edward-bosiljevac-jr-md-phd-facs/

https://www.linkedin.com/pulse/personal-maintenance-reversibility-bosiljevac-jr-md-phd-facs/?trackingId=1UPb%2F%2BUy nansYf3R2REz2A%3D%3D

https://www.linkedin.com/pulse/ozone-oxygen-therapy-coronavirus-bosiljevac-jr-md-phd-facs/?trackingId=t5aT-LOXbNlkPTkBGAuXHKA%3D%3D

https://nypost.com/2020/05/09/new-york-mom-with-coronavirus-saved-by-medical-student-son/?utm_campaign=iphone_nyp&utm_source=mail_app

https://www.ibtimes.com/coronavirus-treatment-cannabis-enzymes-could-help-block-gateway-covid-19-study-2979422

https://www.ibtimes.com/coronavirus-treatment-cannabis-enzymes-could-help-block-gateway-covid-19-study-2979422

54

Aspects Beyond Masks

- **The big deal is a lockdown.**
- **This is not an apocalyptic virus.**
- **After this may be something more severe—this is preparation to be ready.**
- **Dogs can be trained in one week.**
- **The facilities close for the day. A dog cleanup crew is simple and effective.**
- **Anyone with a background in business can start a dog surveillance system.**
- **Avoid a shutdown—that hurt us a lot.**

Lockdown!

The big concern as far as reopening our economy has to do with controlling spread of the virus. This particularly concerns large public facilities, churches, schools, theaters, and also bars and restaurants.

Social distancing has been the key for us with closure of

indoor activities and an enclosed environment.

How does society manage this? Ultraviolet lights may be used in large buildings or the subway, for instance, to disinfect. I have pointed out previously the use of dogs. This current article (see link at end of chapter) reinforces the usefulness of dogs. They are trained in about a week. They can detect areas of concentration that needs particularly better disinfection.

Dogs can be used to screen people before entering a large public facility. They can be used afterwards to help focus on areas of cleanliness. I have mentioned this before.

Think in terms of how many patients have been told by their doctors not to eat red meat. This had nothing to do with whether the beef was grass fed or feedlot and corn fed. That is the real key if the red meat is healthy.

At the suggestion to avoid red meat, attention turns to eating chicken. Have you ever seen photographs of a farm that commercially raises eggs or meat?

The coronavirus is a cousin to the avian or bird flu virus.

The bird flu in chickens may present as a future apocalyptic virus.

There are rumors that this coronavirus was genetically engineered by the Chinese to push an economic standstill on our country. My comment is that in the future an apocalyptic pandemic may originate from somewhere else in the world. This could be a bird or pig (porcine) virus. Both of these can be spread to humans (zoonotic virus). Right now, source is not important. Our response as a society to the pandemic and measures to improve personal hygiene and health are essential for long-term survival.

From the social aspect there are dogs and ultraviolet light

for surveillance and disinfection. Social distancing and masks are also important during an epidemic.

The rest of the key is personal hygiene and improving health overall.

PERSPECTIVE

I was walking to the office one afternoon and I saw a Hispanic man and two Latin women standing by a van. The women would go down the streets with bags to collect recyclables such as plastics, glass, and cans. The man stayed with the truck and loaded recyclables as they were collected.

I like to practice my Spanish, so I went up and spoke to the gentleman. He was originally from Ecuador. They would go daily to parts of the city where recyclables from apartment buildings were placed on the sidewalk for pickup.

After four hours of working and collecting recyclables how much money did they make? He told me $40 is a good day. This encounter helps me understand the struggles other people have with life. At least the recyclables continue as an income source when employment is difficult. The system works well despite a concentrated population. People keep discarding and recycling.

Furthermore, for eight years I had three dogs in Manhattan. Over the years the dogs and I visited most parts of Central Park and other areas of Manhattan. There would be two daily walks. In the morning we would go to Central Park and in the afternoon walk along the East River. In Central Park from six until nine in the morning the dogs could be off leashes. This is where they wore themselves out trying to catch squirrels.

Three years ago, my mother became very ill and I needed to leave New York to be with her for over a month. To board the dogs was $150 a night. I found a farm in Pennsylvania and they are all there now playing in the country. The encounter on the sidewalk with the people doing recyclables occurred during one of the afternoon dog walks. This is a good memory for me.

T-CELL IMMUNITY IN CORONAVIRUS INFECTIONS

I am going to keep the science aspect at the lay level. I think it is important to understand some of these principles because many patients feel that all the information is available and valid. We are still learning how to deal with this pandemic.

There is the personal health aspect related to suffering an infection. Another aspect is social which includes hygiene. The last is availability of testing, ultraviolet lights for disinfection, and other things that may be useful in controlling a pandemic.

T cells are part of the immune system. They are primarily produced in the thymus gland. This is a small gland that is about the size of a couple of almonds and is located under the breastbone around the windpipe. T cells are killers.

It takes time for antibodies to form. If the patient is highly resistant from prior virus infections, then the T cells could respond very quickly as a rapid body defense. T cells can act as a killer cell, a helper when another cell like a macrophage is attacking a microorganism, and the T cell also has a memory. T cells can remember and kill off the virus. This memory may persist.

We were formally taught in medical school that the T cell is a killer cell and a B cell is one that has memory for producing antibodies. Obviously, the way we are put together demonstrate some matching and interchangeable characteristics. This is my point about the body healing itself as the most direct course to promote health. In some patients the T cells are ready to fight immediately. The patient does not get a significant infection and may not form antibodies.

T cell characteristics are important as far as our immunity. It is also a very reliable marker of previous exposure and immunity. There has been a lot of discussion with the coronavirus over antibody testing. T cell immunity is different than antibody formation.

To perform this test for T cell immunity is not feasible for large scale use at this time. It is also expensive. However, this can be a start to develop a more promising test to help understand better the dynamics of this epidemic.

Curcumin has tremendous antiviral qualities. Here is a list of human pathogens against which curcumin has been shown (mostly in vitro) to exhibit antiviral effects:

- Hepatitis B virus
- Hepatitis C virus
- Human papillomavirus, (the cause of genital warts that may lead to malignant squamous cell cervical cancers)
- Dengue virus (mosquito-borne virus)
- Zika virus (mosquito-borne virus)
- Chikungunya virus (mosquito-borne virus)
- Japanese encephalitis (an infection of the brain)
- Human respiratory syncytial virus (RSV, a disease that's highly lethal to children under 5)

- Rift Valley fever (a disease that spreads from animals to humans)
- Herpes simplex
- Coxsackieviruses (viruses that may cause hand, food, and mouth disease, as well as diseases of muscles, lungs, and the heart)
- Human immunodeficiency virus (AIDS)
- Influenza viruses PR8, H1N1, and H6N1

Curcumin combined with piperine (black pepper extract) increases absorption.

Again, I point out another example that we are learning general things about medicine that may be used for treating other illnesses. We have very little experience handling a pandemic. We are still learning. Now I also throw out some information regarding a peptide.

The body contains large proteins that are responsible for biologic activity and healing throughout the human organism. It is now feasible to extract small pieces of these large bio proteins which results in a short protein called a peptide. Where the large bio protein has the ability to assist with many biologic functions, the small peptide may have a very specific biologic activity. The following is a good example.

TB 500 will actually stimulate the thymus gland. This will activate T cells for a rapid defense response. In this manner it is boosting the immune system with this viral pandemic.

An interesting aspect about the TB 500 is it can also help to increase thinning hair. I have two gentlemen that after using this for three months for prevention of coronavirus infection indicated that the thickness of their hair had improved.

Other peptides will be introduced in a forthcoming chapter.

https://www.ft.com/content/5cf2ee49-df7a-4990-b337-860cf7737b2f

https://www.independent.co.uk/news/health/coronavirus-immunity-test-t-cell-antibody-community-a9625811.html

https://medicalxpress.com/news/2020-08-exposure-common-cold-coronaviruses-immune.html

https://www.t-nation.com/supplements/the-best-hope-to-prevent-treat-respiratory-viruses

55

Hydration

- **What is hydration? Think of water as well as trace minerals.**
- **Unprocessed water should have a liquid crystalline structure.**
- **The goal is to get water inside the cell.**
- **The structure of water can affect transport that allows proper hydration of cells.**
- **Proper hydration requires transport of trace minerals into and out of cells.**
- **Destruction of water structure can occur in the presence of electronic and other energy waves—where is your cell phone right now? How about the microwave?**
- **There are ways to measure the tissue state of hydration with a reliable office exam.**

Everybody talks about being well hydrated. "Doc, I drink 6

L of water every day."

This is not about the amount of water ingested. This is about balance and transfer of the water through the cell membrane. Hydration is much more than drinking water. The amount of urine is not enough to indicate that hydration status is good. A dry mouth may not be present with chronic dehydration. Dehydration can be very subtle and occur slowly. <u>Intracellular</u> hydration is what is most important as far as overall health.

Babies are 90% body weight water. As adults, we are 70% body weight water. Dehydration increases with age. When cells develop a level of dehydration they do not function properly. This leads to chronic degenerative changes associated with aging and even cancer.

1. The main problem is that the water structure is disorganized after processing.
2. Osmosis attempts to transfer solvents into or out of the water. This can include trace minerals.
3. Filtered water diminishes trace elements as well as removing the contaminants. This processing is the difference between hard and soft water. Having trace minerals in the water is how we assimilate these into our system, and this can include absorption during a shower. Lack of trace minerals is frequently present.
4. It is best if the pH or acid / base balance in the body is on the alkaline side rather than acid. The body is like a glass flask and will balance pH in all the fluid in the flask depending on what is going on in the complete system. Drinking alkaline water does not necessarily make you alkaline. It also depends what else is already

in the flask— including what you eat. Alkaline water does not absorb better.

5. Hydrogen water would be more helpful for overall hydration.

The two parts of hydration are water and trace minerals. First start with **water**. Glass is a very viscous or thick liquid and is formed by a crystalline structure. This allows transparency through the glass. Water should also form a good liquid crystalline structure. What do I mean by this?

This can be measured in different ways. Sometimes the angle of the molecular connection between the oxygen and hydrogen in the water molecule can affect how water molecules interact with each other. If the phase angle is appropriate this allows the water molecules to align into a nice crystalline structure. Hydrating at the cellular level. This structure enables passage of the water and minerals into the cell. Acid-base levels or pH, electrical conduction, and even magnetic fields can potentially affect the crystalline structure of the water. 5 G may be a potential problem—a recent study shows it causes viruses to mutate. It may also affect water structure.

This is not simply a matter of buying spring water or purified water. Source, preparation, transportation, and contaminants may be involved with aspects that could affect the health benefit of water. Certainly, municipal processed water is completely disorganized. As such, it has a decreased ability to penetrate cells and transport substances back and forth.

Think about the whole food concept as far as diet. Nutrient content can be deficient after processing whole food into a box or a can. Processed food is not healthy. What I refer to above is **processed water** when structure is changed. It is a process that can occur in healthy water stored in plastic bottles, for example.

There are many ways to process water. The municipal facility gets things started, and then at home it may be filtered, or undergo an alkaline or osmosis process. Or it can be oxygenated with ozone. Stored water is usually in a plastic bottle.

There is an office exam that is known as an oligoscan that involves using an infrared light ray focused into your hand. Several sample points are analyzed. The light enters the skin and, depending on different minerals, may reflect, absorb, or scatter the light signal. The reflective signal is picked up by the scanner to give tissue levels of minerals as well as heavy metals.

At the end of the oligoscan report are certain mineral ratios. If you were to look at the report, the black line running down the center represents the median. Green color above or below this range would be in the normal range. We are looking at tissue levels of these minerals. Yellow would be on the edge, and red as an outlier. See below.

Bilan Minéraux

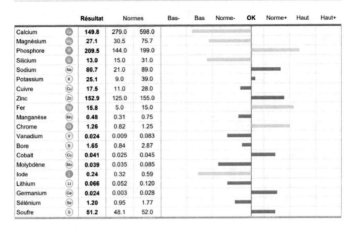

		Résultat	Normes		Bas-	Bas	Norme-	OK	Norme+	Haut	Haut+
Calcium		**149.8**	279.0	598.0							
Magnésium		**27.1**	30.5	75.7							
Phosphore		**209.5**	144.0	199.0							
Silicium		**13.0**	15.0	31.0							
Sodium		**80.7**	21.0	89.0							
Potassium		**25.1**	9.0	39.0							
Cuivre		**17.5**	11.0	28.0							
Zinc		**152.9**	125.0	155.0							
Fer		**15.8**	5.0	15.0							
Manganèse		**0.48**	0.31	0.75							
Chrome		**1.26**	0.82	1.25							
Vanadium		**0.024**	0.009	0.083							
Bore		**1.65**	0.84	2.87							
Cobalt		**0.041**	0.025	0.045							
Molybdène		**0.039**	0.035	0.085							
Iode		**0.24**	0.32	0.59							
Lithium		**0.066**	0.052	0.120							
Germanium		**0.024**	0.003	0.028							
Sélénium		**1.20**	0.95	1.77							
Soufre		**51.2**	48.1	52.0							

Equilibre minéral

Importance des carences
mauvais: 100%

Importance des excès
bon: 60%

319

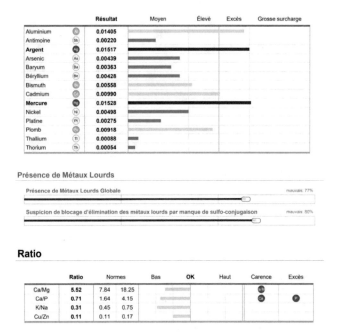

		Résultat	Moyen	Élevé	Excès	Grosse surcharge
Aluminium		0.01405				
Antimoine	(Sb)	0.00220				
Argent	(Ag)	0.01517				
Arsenic	(As)	0.00439				
Baryum	(Ba)	0.00363				
Béryllium	(Be)	0.00428				
Bismuth		0.00558				
Cadmium		0.00990				
Mercure	(Hg)	0.01528				
Nickel	(Ni)	0.00498				
Platine	(Pt)	0.00275				
Plomb		0.00918				
Thallium	(Tl)	0.00088				
Thorium	(Th)	0.00054				

Présence de Métaux Lourds

Présence de Métaux Lourds Globale	mauvais: 77%

Suspicion de blocage d'élimination des métaux lourds par manque de sulfo-conjugaison	mauvais: 80%

Ratio

	Ratio	Normes		Bas	OK	Haut	Carence	Excès
Ca/Mg	**5.52**	7.84	18.25				●	
Ca/P	**0.71**	1.64	4.15				●	●
K/Na	**0.31**	0.45	0.75					
Cu/Zn	**0.11**	0.11	0.17					

Review the oligoscan report as it detects mineral levels within the human machine.

Macronutrients are present in large quantities in our body. Examples are calcium, magnesium, sodium, iron, and potassium. Trace elements would be chromium, iodine, and selenium. The oligoscan helps direct recommendations for supplements for each individual patient.

For instance, sugar metabolism may be poor when chromium is low. Chromium improves insulin sensitivity. Selenium is protective against cancer. If iodine levels are low and there is trouble with thyroid function, treating this by taking additional iodine as a supplement rather than thyroid hormone may be an appropriate first step.

Toxic heavy metals can be detected.

Using this instrument for eight years, I have found it reliable and consistent. Following patients with serial scans can identify which direction patients are moving on their health program.

Look at the **K/Na ratio on the second page**. This stands for the potassium /sodium ratio and reflects the balance of intra-and extracellular water and mineral content. A low number indicates poor intracellular hydration status. Many times, chronic dehydration is corrected by using trace minerals rather than taking more water. This can be demonstrated on serial scans. Using hydrogen water, I have improved my intracellular hydration. Progress can be monitored using the oligoscan.

SALT

I emphasize <u>natural</u> rather than processed salt. Sea salt is processed in most instances and is not a good natural source. Natural salt contains sodium chloride but also trace minerals that work together synergistically with the salt. The ingestion of water <u>alone</u> has little to do with overall hydration. Many of the trace minerals that are present in Himalayan or bamboo salt <u>increase the transport</u> of water into the cell itself and serve the very important aspect to prevent intracellular dehydration.

Himalayan salt is a good option as far as salt containing minerals. Let me give you another option. **Bamboo salt** is prepared in tropical nations by filling fresh bamboo stalks with sea salt.

These are then roasted slowly which leaches trace elements from the bamboo stalk. Differences in bamboo salt result from roasting once or multiple times. Bamboo salt contains crystals of blue and silver (copper, manganese, germanium, and other trace elements) sprinkled throughout the salt. The more roasting the better. Bamboo Salt is Science.

Sea salt has been processed and carries no significant trace minerals. None of the types of salt mentioned contain any significant iodine.

So there is **water** and there are **minerals** and the state of adequate hydration means that everything is in balance. Natural salt is a big part of this. Besides loss of minerals with processing of water the problem can be aggravated by lack of availability in the local environment.

Without trace minerals present during food production the products are lacking in nutrition. This can occur in organic food and there may also be regional differences. An example is that in Israel and Turkey the boron concentrations in the environment are high. There is no problem with low bone density or arthritis in these regions.

Hydration status can improve on a program ingesting less water but supplying certain minerals.

Many things around us in the environment affect the status of water or food. Chemicals can also affect the hydration status. Microwave ovens destroy the integrity and crystalline structure of the water. This can affect the nutritional value of the food cooked in a microwave. We may be out of the "exposure area" of the microwave but the effects are with us in the food. These are new areas of toxicity. High tech detox.

I look at this article as an Introduction to Biophysics and how this affects our health. A very subtle influence.

There are many energy sources such as light, heat, ultrasound, electromagnetic waves, and others known or yet unknown at this time. These energy sources can affect biologic activity in the cell affecting overall function of the "human machine." Medical treatment for conditions caused by these energy sources will become more common in medicine. 5G may be a big one. Look out for phones. A recent study indicated 5G mutates virus. It may also affect the crystalline structure of water.

The bottom line is an unprocessed water source and a system to restore and maintain proper trace minerals into your system. Again, just taking a teaspoon of Himalayan salt may not be sufficient if the water source is not proper. Drinking a ton of processed water alone is meaningless to produce good hydration.

****

A high school social studies teacher presented me with the historical facts below. My comment—the water may have been healthier than what many people drink today—just don't drink after the baby's bath! Also, think about the exposure to minerals from the dirt floor. That could also have been healthy.

Most people got married in June because they took their **yearly bath in May** and so they still smelled pretty good by June. However, since they may be starting to smell...brides carried a bouquet of flowers to hide the body odor. Now we have the custom of carrying **a bouquet** when getting married.

Baths consisted of a big tub filled with hot water. The man of the house had the privilege of the nice clean water, then all the sons and men of the house, then the women, and finally the children. Last of all were the babies. By then the water was so dirty you could actually lose someone in it. Hence the saying "**Don't throw the baby out with the bathwater**!"

There was nothing to stop things from falling into the house with a thatched roof. This posed a natural problem in the bedroom where bugs and other droppings could mess up your nice clean bed. Hence, a bed with big posts and a sheet hanging over the top afforded some protection. That's how **canopy beds** came into existence.

The floor was dirt. Only the wealthy had something other than dirt. Hence the saying "**dirt poor**." The wealthy had slate floors that would get slippery in the winter when wet so they spread straw (thresh) on the floor to help the footing. As the winter wore on, they added more straw (thresh) until when you open the door it would all start slipping outside. A piece of wood was placed on the entrance way. Hence, we have **the threshold**.

http://www.thealternativedaily.com/top-4-reasons-always-tap-water-tested/?utm_source=internal&utm_medium=email&utm_c

https://www.aqualiv.com/the-truth-about-alkaline-water-ionizers-common-misconceptions-about-ph

http://www.thealternativedaily.com/microplastics-in-sea-salt/?utm_source=internal&utm_medium=email&utm_campaign=N151211

http://cenegenics-drbosiljevac.com/?s=lemon+himalayan+salt

https://www.linkedin.com/pulse/dirty-salt-joseph-edward-bosiljevac-jr-md-phd-facs/?trackingId=AK%2FpwKeGmY%2FyZM‹

56

Hydrogen Water

Keep these things in mind. Intracellular hydration is balance inside the cell. Similar to food, water can be processed.

First start with **water**. Glass is a very viscous or thick liquid and is formed as a crystalline structure. This allows transparency through the glass. Water should also form a good liquid crystalline structure. What do I mean by this?

This can be measured in different ways. Sometimes the angle of the molecular connection between the oxygen and hydrogen in the water molecule can affect how water molecules interact with each other. If the phase angle is appropriate this allows the water molecules to align into a nice crystalline structure. Hydrating at the cellular level, This structure enables easy passage of the water and minerals into the cell. Acid-base levels or pH, electrical conduction, and even magnetic fields can potentially affect the crystalline structure of the water. 5 G may be a potential problem—a recent study shows it causes viruses to mutate but I am concerned about the detrimental effect on the structure of water.

To evaluate the effectiveness of water first look if the water has been processed and then evaluate if trace minerals are available. Most water consumed is municipally processed, filtered, and bottled in plastic, all of which can degrade the water structure and content.

Currently there has been an increasing interest in hydrogen water with respect to increasing proper hydration inside the cell.

In this particular case the simplicity of the use of hydrogen water with an overall systemic benefit is quite high. To keep things simple many times gives better results.

The Krebs cycle (to create energy for the cell) shows that the NAD coenzyme uses hydrogen atoms directly to do the work.

1. Water, which is a combination of one oxygen and two hydrogen atoms, has a dissolved portion of hydrogen gas in the water in the concentration of about 0.6 ppm (parts per million). This is the normal status of unprocessed water. Nobody has touched it yet. After processing, it degrades further. Many times, the amount of dissolved hydrogen in processed water we drink is in the range of 0.08 ppm.

2. Most water we all drink to "keep hydrated" is WORTH-LESS—well, let me say significantly suboptimal. Natural water has a normal crystalline structure that enables many of the electromagnetic properties of our body. This structure degrades with processing of water. It also degrades with environmental electromagnetic influences such as cell phones. Very subtle but this can affect our biologic function. The majority of water

we drink is suboptimal to promote healing - actually, it barely sustains us. It slowly degrades and requires considerable energy to restore the normal crystalline structure of water. That's right, you're <u>getting older</u> is accepted. Hydrogen helps us rebuild the crystalline structure of water—that is on the bottom line to restore longevity.

3. Therapeutic effects of hydrogen water has been demonstrated by the Japanese since 2007. It is absorbed through the intestines within one minute and spreads through the entire body in ten. Hydroxyl (-OH) and lipid radicals are erased.

4. There are magnesium tablets that can be dropped into a bottle of water that increase the part per million (ppm) concentration of hydrogen dissolved in water. Some companies claim their product can increase the concentration to 10 ppm. Bottled prepared hydrogen water is not as potent, maybe more the range of 1-2 ppm.

5. If you look at my K/Na ratio I show mild intracellular dehydration with the ratio of 0.31. I have eight years data. This never increased even though I was ingesting more water. I began drinking 3 or 4 of 8-ounce glasses of hydrogen water daily. I prepared this with tablets that make a concentration of 10 ppm dissolved hydrogen in the water. The dissolved hydrogen will make the water opaque. If it is drunk immediately it is absorbed from the intestine within one minute and diffuses throughout the body over 10 minutes. If left alone the opaque water will become clear again as the hydrogen evaporates. Over 2 years my K/Na ratio

improved to 0.45.

6. Is it valid? Yes, and I speak from the aspect of improving the natural ability of the body to function better and heal itself using water that has increased dissolved hydrogen. Look at the detoxification of oxidized radicals. The -OH group encounters a hydrogen atom (H) and forms water (H_2O). Hydrogen serves to detoxify oxidized lipid radicals as well as chemicals and preservatives like hydrogen sulfide in processed food. Reboot. Personal maintenance.

Trace minerals play a part in digestion, blood sugar control, muscle cramps, sleep, and dental health. In addition, they will help with intracellular hydration so that the whole machine is working better. Minerals will be covered next to complete the aspect of hydration.

TYPICAL NYC

I made a home visit to one of my rockstar patient who lives in the Trump World Tower building next to the United Nations. The apartment is on the 35th floor. I noted in the elevator that the top floor was 90. When I commented that the building had 90 floors the patient told me to look at the keypad in the elevator. On my way out I saw many floors missing on the keypad. For example, going from floor 27 the next one was 33. The building actually has only 70 stories instead of the advertised 90.

Ah!!!

New York City. And there are more here besides Trump.

https://www.linkedin.com/pulse/dehydration-ii-joseph-edward-bosiljevac-jr-md-phd-facs/?trackingId=hp53qCu-jYnWwO5uRGl8XFQ%3D%3D

https://www.linkedin.com/pulse/5-g-technology-safe-joseph-edward-bosiljevac-jr-md-phd-facs/?trackingId=hTLzBABqMj

http://www.thealternativedaily.com/microplastics-in-sea-salt/?utm_source=internal&utm_medium=email&utm_campaign=N151211

www.molecularhydrogeninstitute.com

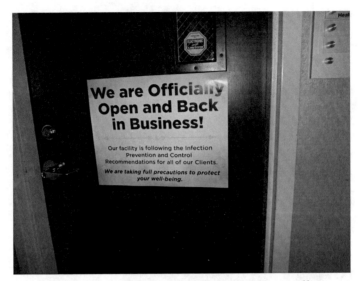

The sign on the front of my office, one we are all too familiar with these days.

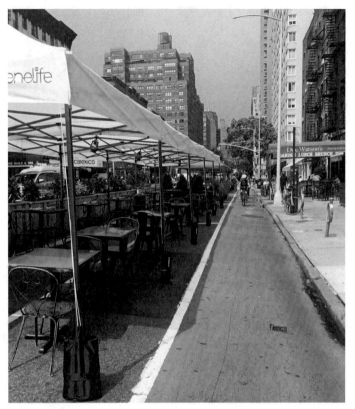

Restaurants are seating patrons on the street to keep revenues high enough to stay open.

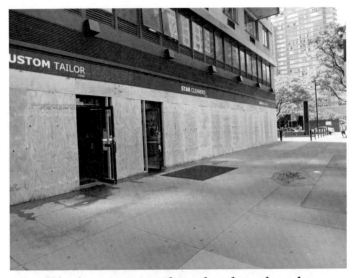

*Small businesses protect themselves from the unknown
intensity of recent protests.*

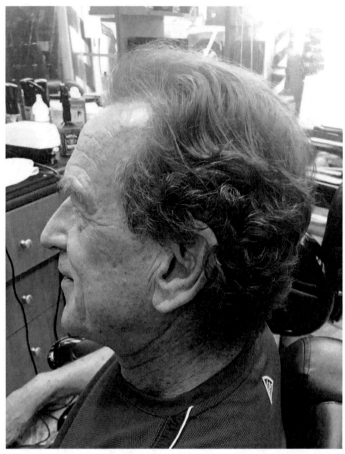

Natural wavy hair after four months sheltering at home in the Upper East Side of Manhattan. July 20, 2020.

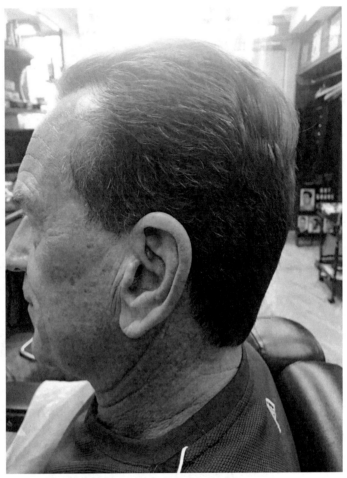

My barber got a good Yelp review after this nicely groomed haircut coming out of quarantine. I have a few grey hairs and he told me he couldn't do anything about my face.

57

Mineral Deficiencies of Modern People

- **Malnutrition can affect us through diet, water, and vitamin and mineral imbalances.**
- **Salt is truly essential to our health.**
- **Bamboo salt is a very nutritious product.**
- **Replacement of trace minerals can actually reverse chronic dehydration.**
- **Subtle and slow changes many times lead to premature aging.**
- **My goal – how at about age 60 you feel "I am only halfway through my life."**

Malnutrition is frequently found in poor Third World countries. My contention is that we have subtle malnutrition going on in our country which aggravates aging.

Besides a low glycemic aspect, I have always promoted the whole food concept as far as <u>diet</u>. This means you do not leave the grocery store with any boxes, cans, packages, or bottles. I have patients tell me "Gee, Doc, then I will not have any groceries."

Good water continues to be a problem. Dehydration is not just lack of water. When we are newborns we are 90% water weight. This is 70% as adults. Then with aging cellular hydration continues to drop. This eventually leads to a chronic or degenerative condition or cancer when the cell cannot respond in a healthy manner. Much of the so-called purified water available has the crystalline structure disorganized. This leads to water that is not as useful to us.

The ingestion of water alone is only part of overall hydration. Many of the trace minerals that are present in Himalayan or bamboo salt increase the transport of water into the cell itself. Salt is a very important aspect to prevent intracellular dehydration.

The quality of our food can be short on vitamin and mineral content. Many **trace minerals** may be absent or depleted depending on the environmental source and location.

In his recent book called Plant Paradox, Dr. Gundry cites a statement from the FDA that the "nutritional aspect of our current growing environment is depleted or very nearly depleted at this time." Most nutrition books talk about a food and associated vitamin and mineral content, which may be much lower than anticipated depending on source of the product. Dr. Gundry points out the importance of source, something not commonly covered in many nutrition books.

Grass fed beef is entirely different than corn fed. Same for dairy products. Farm raised fish is not the same as wild fish. Again, we are talking about additives, preservatives, hormones, and antibiotics that are used with the animal during growth. Dr.

Gundry also points out that the FDA statement above is from 1936. Where are we today?

The continued toxic attack from the environment causes early decline of hormones in our system leading to premature aging. Trace minerals are as key to our health as optimizing hormone levels. And there may be many with low trace mineral levels to the point it affects overall health. The effects are subtle.

The orthodox view in medicine has always been that salt is bad for us. Salt is essential for our health. True salt is not just sodium. Processed salt is not healthy - it contains no trace minerals. Sea (solar) salt and Himalayan salt contain higher potassium and magnesium levels than processed salt. Our body needs these minerals to be healthy.

Attached is a short booklet regarding bamboo salt. Bamboo Salt is Science. The preparation and production of a healthy salt product is reviewed. Poured into your hand you can actually see little colored crystals mixed in with the salt. Basics are presented in this reference article as far as bio physiology and the use of trace minerals for health.

Bamboo salt involves reduction rather than oxidation as far as chemical reactions. Look at the section of photos as far as the reduction and oxidation of nails in certain salt solutions. Chlorine disinfection leads to elevated hypochlorite levels in processed water. A difference is shown between the activity in bamboo salt solution compared to solar and refined (processed) salt solutions to detoxify bad effects of chlorine.

Our exposure of this is not only at the drinking faucet but also includes the shower.

Himalayan and bamboo salt increase the transport of water into the cell itself. Natural salt (actually associated trace minerals) is a very important aspect to prevent intracellular dehydration.

Himalayan salt is a good natural source of salt and contains a variety of trace minerals.

Himalayan salt contains helpful trace elements such as vanadium and germanium. Copper and silica are very important for collagen formation. Platinum is a catalyst for many chemical reactions that promote biosynthesis and assimilation of other trace minerals.

Trace minerals may help with skin and hair conditions. Some systemic conditions such as diabetes and insulin resistance may be improved with chromium. Keep in mind that deficiencies may not cause acute changes or lead to a visit to the emergency room. Changes are subtle and take time.

Additional copper may prevent premature graying of hair. So instead of stress causing gray hair it may really be the subtle loss of trace minerals. What is interesting is the accepted dietary range of the minerals. For the effect on graying of the hair, it may require 4 to 6 mg of copper daily. My family came from Croatia and had lived in an area with a high copper level. Men in the family did not get gray until their seventies. Copper has a lot to do with immunity and thyroid function. It also preserves vision.

Add Epsom salt (magnesium) and Himalayan salt together. After shampooing your hair allow this to soak into the hair and scalp. Let it sit five minutes during the rest of your shower. This keeps your hair thicker and also helps gray go away. I am pushing 70 and I have thick hair and minimal gray.

The copper dose is well above the so-called daily requirement. As far as maximum dose the current reference ranges may not be accurate. Overall, we may be ingesting poor water and lack sufficient trace minerals.

Note that sea salt and bamboo salt do not contain any significant iodine. There is a big misunderstanding for Americans who feel they get iodine out of sea salt since the majority of them still have a significant iodine deficit.

When patients replace trace minerals the dehydration improves. Patients with a history of high blood pressure can actually see numbers come down. Not as much water will need to be ingested. The other gray area here is that it *should be* good water, as noted earlier.

Whole food, organized water, and natural salt are true keys to proper nutrition. With this routine, maybe you do not have to take so many supplements.

We can revisit an office exam called an oligoscan that effectively evaluates and follows tissue levels of minerals. View the sample scan below:

Bilan Minéraux

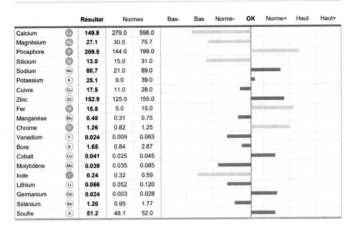

		Résultat	Normes		Bas-	Bas	Norme-	OK	Norme+	Haut	Haut+
Calcium		149.8	279.0	598.0							
Magnésium		27.1	30.5	75.7							
Phosphore		209.5	144.0	199.0							
Silicium		13.0	15.0	31.0							
Sodium		80.7	21.0	89.0							
Potassium		25.1	9.0	39.0							
Cuivre		17.5	11.0	28.0							
Zinc		152.9	125.0	155.0							
Fer		15.8	5.0	15.0							
Manganèse		0.48	0.31	0.75							
Chrome		1.26	0.82	1.25							
Vanadium		0.024	0.009	0.083							
Bore		1.65	0.84	2.87							
Cobalt		0.041	0.025	0.045							
Molybdène		0.039	0.035	0.085							
Iode		0.24	0.32	0.59							
Lithium		0.066	0.052	0.120							
Germanium		0.024	0.003	0.028							
Sélénium		1.20	0.95	1.77							
Soufre		51.2	48.1	52.0							

Equilibre minéral

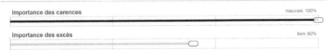

Importance des carences — mauvais: 100%

Importance des excès — bon: 60%

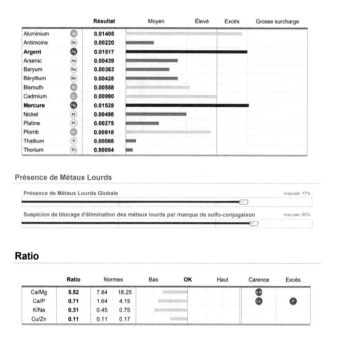

		Résultat	Moyen	Élevé	Excès	Grosse surcharge
Aluminium		0.01405				
Antimoine	(Sb)	0.00220				
Argent		0.01517				
Arsenic	(As)	0.00439				
Baryum	(Ba)	0.00363				
Béryllium	(Be)	0.00428				
Bismuth		0.00558				
Cadmium		0.00990				
Mercure		0.01528				
Nickel	(Ni)	0.00498				
Platine	(Pt)	0.00275				
Plomb		0.00918				
Thallium	(Tl)	0.00088				
Thorium	(Th)	0.00054				

Présence de Métaux Lourds

Présence de Métaux Lourds Globale — mauvais: 77%

Suspicion de blocage d'élimination des métaux lourds par manque de sulfo-conjugaison — mauvais: 80%

Ratio

	Ratio	Normes		Bas	OK	Haut	Carence	Excès
Ca/Mg	5.52	7.84	18.25				●	
Ca/P	0.71	1.64	4.15				●	●
K/Na	0.31	0.45	0.75					
Cu/Zn	0.11	0.11	0.17					

Notice the amount of mineral balance measured inside the body.

This office or bedside exam uses an infrared light to look at levels of about 20 different trace minerals and additionally a dozen heavy metals. The light enters the skin focused into your hand. Several sample points are analyzed and depending on different minerals, may reflect, absorb, or scatter the light signal. The reflective signal is picked up by the scanner to give tissue levels of minerals as well as heavy metals.

It measures **tissue levels (not a blood or urine test)**. The exam is accurate and consistent when followed in a serial fashion. The oligoscan collects objective data on mineral balance to assess if supplements or other treatment are being effective. We are looking at specific data points to help us evaluate overall balance of the human machine.

As you look at the report, the black line running down the center represents the median. Again, we are talking about tissue levels of these minerals so green color above or below this range would be in the normal range. Yellow would be on the edge, and red as an outlier.

Macronutrients are present in large quantities in our body. Examples are calcium, magnesium, sodium, iron, and potassium. Trace elements would be chromium, iodine, and selenium. The oligoscan helps direct recommendations for supplements for each individual patient.

Trace minerals serve an important part in many biologic activities. Trace elements and minerals can have a complex relationship with each other. Zinc relates with copper which also boosts the immune system. Significant biologic changes can be affected but symptoms of deficiency may be so subtle that no one needs to go to the emergency room.

Trace mineral deficiencies can also affect intracellular hydration. Minerals work with water as far as balanced, effective movement inside and outside of cells. I am not convinced that current medical reference ranges are not optimal many times including recommendations for supplemental intake.

Trace minerals may be depleted or absent from plants or produce because of depletion in the surrounding environment. The appropriate food is eaten, but the nutritional value is suboptimal. I repeat the following:

In his recent book called <u>Plant Paradox</u>, *Dr. Gundry cites a statement from the FDA that the* **'nutritional aspect of our current growing environment is depleted or very nearly depleted at this time.'** *Most nutrition books talk about a food and associated vitamin and mineral content,* <u>*which may be much lower than anticipated depending on source of the product.*</u> *Dr. Gundry points out the importance of* <u>*source*</u>, *something not commonly covered in many nutrition books.*

Grass fed beef is entirely different than corn fed. Same for dairy products. Farm raised fish is not the same as wild fish. Again we are talking about additives, preservatives, hormones, and antibiotics that are used with the animal during growth. Dr. Gundry also points out that the FDA statement above is from **1936**. *Where are we today?*

Again, consider the scan from above. I have eight years data with this exam. Hard, consistent, objective data is frequently missed in the usual annual physical. And think about blood work. Did you ever hear of a man having a progesterone level drawn? Sometimes this is significant. Data points are used that direct the approach to treatment and allows accurate trending and follow-up. The oligoscan has been essential.

At the end of the <u>oligoscan</u> report are certain mineral ratios. If you look at my K/Na ratio I show mild intracellular dehydration with the ratio of 0.31. This never increased even though I was ingesting more water. I began drinking 3 or 4 of 8-ounce glasses of hydrogen water daily and after <u>two</u> years noted an improvement. See how subtle this is.

As mentioned before, I prepared this with tablets that make a concentration of 10 ppm dissolved hydrogen in the water. The dissolved hydrogen will make the water opaque. If it is drunk immediately it is absorbed from the intestine within one minute and diffuses throughout the body over 10 minutes. If left alone the opaque water will become clear again as the hydrogen evaporates. Over 2 years my K/Na ratio improved to 0.45.

TOXIC AND GOOD HEAVY METALS

The oligoscan can also look at heavy metals. There are good heavy metals such as iodine and selenium. Toxic ones are cadmium, aluminum, mercury, and lead which can adversely affect the immune system and other areas. Although heavy metals may affect an acute illness, many aspects are low key and subtle and not thought to be so important regarding long-term prevention. Low tissue iodine can detrimentally affect levels the function of the thyroid. Persistence of symptoms of a low immune system can be a subtle sign of trace mineral deficiency or heavy metal excess.

I see thyroid deficiency with many of my patients. As patients get older, there are some in whom the thyroid function may be better one day than another. Before they reach a chronic low thyroid level, there is a transition period. In this phase sometimes patients will have hypothyroid like symptoms that are more severe one day and not so bad on other days. Now the key point here is when blood levels are drawn. This may show different levels as far as thyroid function depending on the day the blood is drawn. Sometimes it may or it might correlate with a low thyroid condition. Unless this is kept in mind, many patients with suboptimal thyroid function will be missed in conventional medicine.

It is a challenge to line up and evaluate data to help define a difficult diagnosis. It is not black and white. These things take judgment. I was never taught any of this in medical school. I have had more than 300,000 patient encounters in my clinical career. A lot of my judgment is based on that.

When iodine levels are noted to be low, many times I have noted improved thyroid function in patients with adequate iodine supplementation rather than giving thyroid hormone. Copper and ferritin (iron) deficiency can affect thyroid function.

Note that my iodine levels were on the lower side. My thyroid function bloodwork is normal. I started to supplement iodine to maintain good thyroid function long term.

Most nutrition booklets will state that 250 µg a day should be taken. This is far below what I have found is an adequate dose for iodine with American patients. Over 2 years my iodine levels began to rise with a dose of 3000 micrograms a day. There is nothing toxic about this dose. We are following an optimal personal program instead of relying on the directions on the bottle. Although heavy metals may affect an acute illness, many aspects are low key and subtle and not thought to be so important regarding long-term prevention.

Chromium levels are frequently low in patients with adult onset diabetes and insulin resistance. Supplementation with 800 -1000 µg daily over a one-year time may markedly improve sugar metabolism and diabetes.

Boron is found remotely concentrated in certain areas. Turkey and Israel are part of this area. There is a high incidence of low bone density in the USA and most menopausal women are taking medication for this. In those countries with high boron levels in the environment bone density is normal and there is minimal arthritis. I have seen patients improve their bone density with boron. With bone density medications, the best that can be expected is to maintain the bone density. With boron it can be increased. How about together? Another aspect of bone density has to do with optimal levels of sex hormones. Use boron together along with hormone optimization.

Selenium is important as far as an anticancer effect in the genitourinary system.

Although heavy metals may affect an acute illness, many aspects are low key and subtle and not thought to be so important regarding long-term prevention.

Toxic heavy metals are displayed on the second page of the oligoscan. I have personal and other patient records for eight years and I feel this testing is reliable, consistent, and reproducible to follow progress. Note that the mercury levels are up. I was having some dental work done at that time and I would see my mercury levels go up and then come down over a period of about a month after the dental work. When the dental work was done my mercury levels were still elevated. Mercury is significant for vision and other nerve system conditions.

Some heavy metals are healthy, such as iodine and selenium. How is this relevant?

I have noticed that when patients push the good heavy metals then the toxic heavy metal levels go down. To detoxify from heavy metals does not always require intravenous chelation. I am taking about 3000 µg of iodine and 400 µg of selenium every other day. This is much higher than the recommended dose. There have been no adverse reactions. Over a year of initiating this dose I noted that my mercury levels went down without chelation. Cilantro and chlorophyll in the diet are also helpful to naturally chelate and excrete toxic heavy metals.

With heavy metals (iron is another example) I have noticed that assimilation is better when given on an intermittent rather than daily basis. For this reason, I take 400 mg of the selenium every other day. There is no need to take 20 supplements daily. Depending on diet, intermittent supplementation may promote more favorable benefits.

In my practice I have seen toxic heavy metals that contribute to a chronic problem. Many times, toxic heavy metals are not well understood and are ignored by conventional medicine.

Argent is the French name for silver. The server for the oligoscan is in Paris. Most Americans have silver in the red range. This may be from silverware, jewelry, or maybe watches. I have not seen these levels be toxic or cause a clinical health risk

I once saw a middle-aged lady from Massachusetts. Her arsenic levels were extremely high. However, she stated that when she was growing up as a little girl all the neighbors commented on the high arsenic levels in the well water. This additional data is part of the workup that helps me do better prevention with age management. Arsenic poisoning has many gastrointestinal symptoms. A diagnosis of cancer would make me address this immediately.

Many times, I see with the military special forces high cadmium and antimony levels from firearm use. This can be associated with heat sensitivity—which is something I see in these patients. I also see this affect skin cancer and pancreas cancer.

Aluminum levels are frequently noted to be elevated. Many times, this is due to deodorant that contains aluminum. However, aluminum cookware is so common in the kitchen. I was taught to cook with food wrapped in aluminum foil. The heating of the aluminum allows it to enter into the food and then into us. Can this be enough to promote dementia?

Mercury and cadmium levels appear to be elevated in the Northeast United States because of environmental exposure. I also have done this testing on patients in the Midwest and note that results are different for heavy metal toxicity depending on the region.

Once again, I talk about the use of liposomal encapsulation. EDTA is an agent that binds and allows excretion of toxic heavy metals. It is not well absorbed by mouth and is usually given by the intravenous route. This is not entirely convenient for patients to go in and get chelation twice a week for three months at the doctor's office. Liposomal encapsulation of EDTA allows good absorption. A source I trust is *Quicksilver Scientific*. A clear liposomal solution contains smaller liposomes that are absorbed better. Sublingual is convenient and can be very effective.

When I was doing IV chelation on patients, I measured a 24-hour urine after treatment to see what was being pulled out. Two weeks after the IV chelation I gave a course of liposomal EDTA with several patients. 24-hour urine collection demonstrated similar results as far as excretion of the toxic heavy metals. More convenient and effective. There are no large conventional studies, but current medicine does not believe in chelation anyway.

Heavy metal toxicity may cause subtle signs or changes in our health that many times is not recognized.

Whole food, organized water, and natural salt are true keys to proper nutrition. With this routine, maybe so many supplements are not necessary.

For adequate hydration minimally processed water and trace minerals are essential. We are talking about the ability for these substances to enter into the cell itself. Intracellular hydration is the key.

Chronic intracellular dehydration, extremely low iodine levels, low chromium and selenium levels, and some elevation in toxic heavy metals can all play a significant part in overall health.

Addressing the areas mentioned could add good-quality years to a person's life. That is a concept about preventive health - not only more years, but good ones. Would it not feel good to reach 60 and say "Well, my life is only half over? And, I have no concern with a new pig virus epidemic in the future. We know how to handle this stuff."

How aggressive do you want to be? The first step is getting a significant set of data points to help develop a baseline and give some direction. That is the only decision you need to make for now. That is the first step. Then decide where to go from there.

That is what I do.

http://cenegenics-drbosiljevac.com/blog/is-it-only-water/

http://www.thealternativedaily.com/9-benefits-of-letting-your-kids-play-in-the-dirt/?utm_source=internal&utm_medium=em

58

The Case of the Navy SEAL

From Nick:

I retired from the Navy in 2013 with 28+ years. 25 was as a SEAL. I was dealing with neurological problems. When I went to the Neurologist, I was told I had MS (Multiple Scars). I knew I had numerous TBI's and other injuries, so I didn't think much about having scars. That's normal right? That was all that was said and the other Doctors at the TBI clinic didn't take any history or run additional test or anything additional. This was also the same once I retired.

In 2012 I went on the MS Auto Immune suppressant medication. After 3 years my situation had deteriorated, and I quit taking the AI (Auto Immune) medications that had been destroying my T Cells by design.

I did 40 Hyperbaric Oxygen dives and a lot of the symptoms subsided and I felt better. I did 40 more and felt even better. I did several treatments to help reverse some of the neurological problems I was dealing with to include the MERT system.

By 2018 I had not fully recovered from the neurological and health problems that continued to plague me.

I was positive that the MS, AI medications had shut down my immune system and I was unable to recover, which had left me vulnerable to everything I already had and more.

After a hospital stay in the beginning of 2019, I began looking for additional natural treatments to help me. This is where I met Doctor Bosiljevac and learned through my daughter that he did Stem Cell Therapy. She and a good friend of 30 years set up a fundraiser and I went to see him in New York.

From the day I contacted him, he was very involved in teaching me about how his treatment protocol worked in the body, about my history and how I had felt at different times over the years. He asked questions that I had never been asked before by another doctor. He also gave me a blood panel to have drawn and tested. It was about two pages longer than any other blood panel I had ever been given to include 5 Year Dive Physicals.

Doctor Bosiljevac over the next year gave me a Stem Cell infusion with Umbilical Stem Cells, an injection of Stem Cells into my cranium, Multiple NAD and Exosome IV infusions, a PEPTIDE treatment and Testosterone injections.

The purpose was to promote healing throughout my body and reset my immune system.

Stem Cells do not produce immediate results, but you get results over time and they can be subtle until one day you are like 'wow I feel pretty good' or your pain level is lower or nonexistent. You also have to do what you can to help the Stem Cells do their job and help you, to include:

Taking vitamins and minerals, maintain a healthy diet (I

do the Ketogenic eating habits) to reduce inflammation.

It's been 1 year since I began Doctor Bosiljevac's Stem Cell Protocol and I still feel a little better each day. The numbness in my feet has disappeared, Pain in my feet is 95% gone, I no longer have incontinence, I do not fall down as often because I can feel my foot placement.

He has encouraged me to do MERT again and Hyperbaric Therapy and has monitored my progress and blood work. If I have questions, we email and I have answer within 48 hours or we actually speak over the phone.

Along came COVID-19 and I haven't had a reservation about doing my normal activities. In fact, I have not been sick with a cold or even the sniffles since I began his Stem Cell protocol.

I have just completed a SPECT Scan of my brain. It shows years of trauma injuries to my brain and some from possible heavy metals and exposure. The significant part of this is that it also showed areas that show improvement. The things I have done in the last year has been Hyperbaric Therapy, MERT, BEMER and Doctor Bosiljevac's Stem Cell protocol.

I fully believe that Doctor Bosiljevac's Stem Cell protocol can and will help many people with various injuries and illnesses. This also includes some people who are not getting answers from the medical community. I also believe that it can help with quality of life for those individuals that have no quality of life.

Nick Baggett, 26 July 2020

From Doc Joe:

In my opinion this is all about wound healing. Hyperbaric oxygen is one of those modalities assisting with that. Optimizing hormones will improve the environment for healing and regeneration.

Nick's workup consisted of getting extensive lab work. He was tested for trace minerals, and heavy metals, and also for nitric oxide levels. Cardiovascular testing was done. A dexa scan gave body composition and bone density. At that point we have good data points to direct a game plan to help this patient with recovery.

After his first treatment with IV NAD, Nick was able to walk all the way into the bathroom from his wheelchair. He had not done that for 1 ½ years prior to the treatment.

An interesting aspect is that approximately 90 days following the treatment Nick began to have an increase and recurrence in some of his symptoms. The cycle for stem cells to divide, grow, and differentiate is about 90 days. I have seen this happen many times in autoimmune conditions. When the symptoms recur, the patient is actually returning to a state of health and going through a level of symptoms that developed with their condition. He had a repeat NAD treatment and exosomes with complete loss of symptoms following the treatment. No stem cells were needed.

It is not the stem cells causing these symptoms but the inflammatory effects of the autoimmune condition. I have had patients go to urgent care with these recurrent symptoms and several were told that this is the bad effect of stem cells. Wrong!

Further treatment is necessary in approximately 80% of

patients. What we are doing depends where the individual patient stands as far as wound healing. The availability of exosomes allows continuance of the healing process without having to reintroduce stem cells. Exosomes act as growth factors for all this and to improve overall patient health status and ability to heal.

Healing properly depends on personal health. This program approaches that goal by rebooting cells and rejuvenation. Nick is doing a big part with a keto diet.

When I talked with Nick twelve months following his treatment, he was very pleased with results. There was still some brain scar on a SPEC scan, but this had actually improved. The strength and the painful neuropathy in the legs both improved significantly.

We are not done with his healing. We will know more long-term results after 1 to 2 years. How about the patient's ability to heal?

This is all about wound healing.

The rest of the key is personal hygiene and improving health overall.

Probably 80% of Americans need to be rebooted including many who deny subtle changes.

https://www.linkedin.com/pulse/what-does-mean-reboot-joseph-edward-bosiljevac-jr-md-phd-facs/

https://www.linkedin.com/pulse/personal-maintenance-reversibility-bosiljevac-jr-md-phd-facs/?trackingId=1UPb%2F%2B nansYf3R2REz2A%3D%3D

https://www.linkedin.com/pulse/benefit-rejuvenation-

joseph-edward-bosiljevac-jr-md-phd-facs-1f/?trackingId=Y7x9O8C1
DIJEd0Uuemqg%3D%3D

59

Dialing Down on Health

One night I was up late with paperwork. My girlfriend got off work about midnight. I planned to go out and meet her at the subway. It was hot in the apartment and I took my shirt off and threw it on the bed.

I continued to work and then noticed she had sent a text that she was on the subway. I put the shirt on and rushed to the subway. I am standing there trying to look attentive as she arrived. She came through the gate and started laughing. She told me I was getting to be an old man! I had my shirt on inside out!

I do not exactly remember, but if that is the worst thing I did that day - it was a good day. Besides, I had not seen my girlfriend for a week.

There are always different and remarkable ways presented to promote longevity. Resveratrol, surtuins, peptides like epitalon and other supplements are touted for anti-aging.

My contention is that this needs to start with the basics of normal cell biology and energy production. Biologic chemicals deplete in the cells over time. This is considered 'normal aging.' By rebooting cells of these depleted substances, they can function more optimally. The metabolic function of the human organism improves and wound healing and tissue regeneration is promoted.

These aspects of aging are very subtle. Society says that 'you're just getting older.' There is nothing urgent that makes you go to the emergency room. However, you start on the downward slope.

This article mentions that some cells have a slow decline in the stability of the nucleus and some cells appear to age primarily due to dysfunctional mitochondria. Mitochondria are organelles that produce energy for the cell.

After genetics, which is not changeable, look at lifestyle items to improve longevity.

So, let's take this down to the basics. The nucleus and the mitochondria are the two common areas of cellular decline in function.

As far as the nucleus we are looking at preservation of telomeres and prevention of DNA degradation that may occur with some things such as smoking, x-ray exposure, and other environmental factors.

Take a shoestring and hold it out in front with both hands. This represents a DNA strand. Normally this is accompanied by a second DNA strand and they are wound together in a certain molecular and biologic structure. The little plastic 'aglets' on both ends that protect stability of the DNA (shoestring) during reproduction represent telomeres. Each time the DNA strand replicates, these aglets prevent unraveling of the ends of the DNA strand.

I have promoted the personal maintenance program that actually restores or reboots cells back to more optimal function.

Telomeres are good measurements to reflect biologic age. In this regard telomeres may be preserved or sometimes with the use of a peptide called epitalon may actually increase in length. That makes a patient biologically younger!

I have one patient who eight years ago had a baseline chronological age of 62 and a biologic age of 56 using telomere measurement. A health program for 8 years was followed including a year of epitalon. In follow-up at a chronologic age of 70 the patient's biologic age was 54 using the same telomere measurement. Biologically the same or younger.

As far as mitochondria, look at the Krebs cycle which is basically the source of the energy production in the cell. NAD is a coenzyme that encourages the process. NAD depletes with age. In patients who have chronic neurodegenerative conditions such as multiple sclerosis have nerve cells that have dumped out all the NAD, leading to neuropathies and many other neurologic symptoms.

There is a type of protein involved regulating cellular processes during aging and death of cells and also provide resistance to stress. This is called sirtuin 1 or SIRT 1. These are notably an important part in DNA repair and maintaining metabolic balance in many tissues. They are particularly necessary in the mitochondria. Activating the protein has been shown in various studies to improve overall health benefits including longevity. Their activity is related directly to NAD levels. Resveratrol is one of the supplements that activates sirtuin activity. NAD is an example of mechanisms that start with the basics. This is the key is far as rebooting the system.

Restoration of NAD levels in the cell can improve mitochondrial function and energy production. The cell produces normal energy and everything is good. With decreased energy degenerative symptoms develop, including chronic conditions and even cancer.

So, there are many lifestyle items to look at to improve to a healthy lifestyle. This information emphasizes the need to concentrate on the nucleus as well as the mitochondria. Rebooting cells and rejuvenation.

https://www.linkedin.com/pulse/what-does-mean-reboot-joseph-edward-bosiljevac-jr-md-phd-facs/

https://www.linkedin.com/pulse/personal-maintenance-reversibility-bosiljevac-jr-md-phd-facs/?trackingId=1UPb%2F%2BUy nansYf3R2REz2A%3D%3D

https://www.worldhealth.net/news/has-cellular-aging-master-circuit-been-discovered/

https://www.linkedin.com/pulse/can-you-get-younger-joseph-edward-bosiljevac-jr-md-phd-facs/?trackingId=YpvD-sqqJ80moEutzbWJdzg%3D%3D

https://www.linkedin.com/pulse/therapeutic-use-nad-joseph-edward-bosiljevac-jr-md-phd-facs/?trackingId=9cd-hBG5nwMWj2gV1%2FNskIA%3D%3D

60

Rotting of the Big Apple

World famous monument of George Washington is defaced as NYC city slides billions into the red, its police face $1bn in cuts and de Blasio is accused of 'surrendering the city to lawlessness'

- **The monument at Washington Square Park was defaced on Monday by vandals who threw red paint at it.**
- **President Trump tweeted that it had been defaced by 'anarchists' who would be 'tracked down.'**
- **Downtown, hundreds gathered outside City Hall for an #OccupyCityHall protest ahead of the budget vote.**
- **They say they will not move until the city council strips at least $1billion from the NYPD budget.**
- **They are calling for the NYPD to be defunded; the new budget, expected on Tuesday, strips it of $1billion.**
- **The cut accounts for more than 16% of the force's**

$6billion annual budget but some say it's not enough.

- **It involves a class of 1,163 recruits who were due to graduate in July not being given jobs yet.**
- **The city has a $9billion deficit as a result of the coronavirus pandemic which slashed tax revenues.**
- **NYPD Commissioner Dermot Shea says the $1bn cut is a 'punitive' reaction to the BLM protests.**
- **Unions say Mayor de Blasio is 'surrendering the city to lawlessness' and putting New Yorkers at risk.**
- **Crime is spiking in New York City with shootings and burglaries on the rise.**

By JENNIFER SMITH FOR DAILYMAIL.COM

PUBLISHED: 08:11 EDT, 30 June 2020 | **UPDATED:** 15:33 EDT, 30 June 2020

24 July 2020

Is the city rotting or not? The above article was written one month earlier.

I am a transplanted Midwesterner who began working here in 2008. I have always felt safe in New York City. New York has been the epicenter of the pandemic the last four months. Recent experience trying to ban police and watching various demonstrations and riots now has me more concerned about security in the city. Since I arrived several years after 9/11, I have always felt safe against terrorists. Not right now. Not as much.

There are a lot of mom-and-pop stores closed. I have a small practice in age management that has been dead for four months. My practice is like a mom and pop store. Or maybe a grandpa store since I am pushing 70.

This is like taking a year out of my life—but I am not traveling anywhere. It would be hard to manage kids out of school and work. I am hardly working. The high New York overhead continues.

Restaurants are not making any money serving outside only. Commercially, New York City is very slow.

The Yankees opened the baseball season with the Washington Nationals. Without fans in the stadium this is boring.

Subways have 8 to 10 people per car—25% normal.

Everything is shut down. Large public events, restaurants, and bars continue to be closed.

A decision on opening public schools will be made about 20 days from today.

The city normally has some 60 million tourists every year. There are less people on the sidewalks, in Central Park, and businesses are very slow. It is easier to shop online than go to a store. The city is not getting any taxes. My patients from out of state or out of the country are very reluctant to come to New York City right now.

If this is an engineered viral attack to slow us socially, economically, and with personal health then we need to learn how to handle the pandemic. We also need to work on personal health for resistance and recovery from infection.

An engineered virus could come from another part of the world at any time. The current COVID-19 is not an apocalyptic virus.

Personal maintenance.

STRAND BOOKSTORE – A GLIMMER OF NOR-MALCY

Back in the early 1970s I saw a movie named 'The Reincarnation of Peter Proud' with Michael Sarazin and Jennifer O'Neill.

Later I purchased the book and have read it five or six times over the years.

There is a used bookstore here in Manhattan called Strand Books. They advertise 18 miles of bookshelves in the store. Closed for several months they have now reopened five days a week with limited hours. I went down to see if I could find any other books by the same author, Max Ehrlich.

I found one of his first books written in 1955 named 'First Train to Babylon.' This book focuses on a family in Long Island and is a very good read.

My surprise was that this hardback book was a first edition and this signature was inside the cover.

Sincerely and
With Warm Regards

Max Ehrlich

61

Can This be More Simple?

Early August 2020

I do not want to get into politics but I feel that handling the pandemic can be more simple. Many of the people making decisions already receive a salary and continue to get their pension. For most of them this is no big deal personally. They have not been affected like the general population.

We live in a world with viruses and we need to learn how to survive. Politicians are playing a FEAR game with the public. So this may have been necessary just to get Americans to think about wearing a mask.

Some general comments are presented with my wide background and experience in healthcare for 45 years and living in Manhattan this entire year with the pandemic. I have also been involved with antibody testing of patients.

1. We are dealing with a virus and this should be approached from what we know about viruses in general. A lot of fears are being thrown out as far as recurrence, virulence

(spreading), and mutation of the virus.

Any differences with the coronavirus will be learned with time.

Though this may have been genetically engineered is not significant at this time. It is possible that an apocalyptic virus may be put out by some other country in the future. This coronavirus is not the one yet.

We need to learn from the current pandemic.

2. The best and natural way for survival and resistance to spread is to have the majority of the population exposed and recover with antibodies. This is called **herd immunity**. A vaccine would also promote herd immunity but that is not available today.

We will see some increase in coronavirus incidence as we open society. This should not cause another shut down although politicians are scared that they may lose their job so they drag feet and even go on vacation. Think about the small shop and restaurant owners being told just take a vacation for 6 to 12 months. No income. Most of these are self-employed with limited savings and high overhead.

Providing hygiene, precaution, prevention, and protecting the elderly are key elements.

Herd immunity is the resistance to the spread of a contagious disease that results if a sufficiently high proportion of a population is immune to the illness. At that point, some people are still susceptible but they are surrounded by immune individuals, who serve as a barrier preventing the microbes from reaching them. Herd immunity can be achieved through either mass infection or mass vaccination. Epidemiologists have converged on an estimate that 60 to 70 percent of people need to either have been vaccinated or infected to reach herd immunity for COVID-19.

The current pandemic was handled in Sweden without a complete lockdown. This enabled them to achieve **herd immunity** more quickly.

3. We really do not have any overall statistics regarding prior viral epidemics for comparison. A lot of testing has been done with COVID-19 in New York. Overall, incidence of positive throat cultures occurs in about 0.5% of the population here in the city. There are no statistics as far as spreading of the Asian bird virus. We have no long-term data on how many people are antibody positive with the Asian bird flu. Think about chicken farms.

Attention is paid to positive antibodies in large bird populations that are involved in our food process. This results in many birds culled so they do not enter the food chain. We continue to learn. I say be careful eating chickens from commercial farms.

4. Is this virus worse than the Spanish flu or the Hong Kong flu? Is it more contagious?

At my age, I know Woodstock. Maybe I was there (another story). The coronavirus is a cousin to the avian bird flu virus. Both are zoonotic which means they can spread between animal and person. The coronavirus is associated with a higher death rate, although the mortality rate may be higher due to infection in nursing homes and with high-risk patients because proper measures were not taken initially.

COVID-19 antibody positive findings in Corona, New York (Queens, 23 August) was seen in 68% of patients. In Manhattan it is 19%. The Bronx had 33% antibody positive testing. Remember **herd immunity**.

I was talking with a younger sister who lives in Kansas City. She works in the school system and is concerned because of the increased outbreak of corona in her community. New York is settling down while other parts of the country are beginning to see some increase in infections. This is simply following the course of a viral epidemic. It started in New York. We are a little bit ahead in the game. Other areas will begin to feel some symptoms now. Remember that viruses will become universal when there are humans to spread transmission. There are usual precautionary methods, personal hygiene items, and then some of the preventive measures I note later in this article.

With time the testing data will help see trending based on data collected. Again, we are learning.

5. The concern is spread and how to do this without closing doors and remaining in quarantine forever.

There are questions about what is the virulence of a mutated coronavirus. How long do antibodies last? No one knows. Approach this as other viruses for now and time will give more information as data is gathered and analyzed.

We need to be ready as a country. Americans do not want to be told to wear a mask so we had to learn. Stay home. Stay safe. We are in this together. These are the mantras we have become accustomed to. But this is not the same across the board for everyone.

I recently saw a 17-year-old high school boy who was angry to see that advice. He did not feel his home was safe. He felt safe at school and also with his previous job working at a restaurant. The government officials in charge of the recent choices are not considering the aspects of freedom that our country is founded on. Most importantly, the freedom to make a living for yourself and your family. By taking personal health measures we can move forward with businesses open while still keeping ourselves safe. Living in the world, not waiting for the world to change for us.

How Can It Be More Simple?

A. Personal hygiene with facemasks, increased social distancing, and handwashing is essential.

B. Dogs can be used to monitor coronavirus and direct disinfection. The military has trained dogs within a week.

C. Ultraviolet radiation can be used for disinfection. Shine this at night from each classroom ceiling. This can be used in other public locations such as a restaurant and even the subway, with some restrictions or precautions for exposure with people. Shine them in the subway during the nighttime shutdown.

D. Another personal hygiene item has to do with iodine spray for the nose. The British health system study demonstrated this is an excellent preventive measure since iodine is toxic to viruses.

There is current work to develop a coronavirus breathalyzer test. See the source below for detailed information. These are all just other options to consider going forward so we can function as a society, and not stay stagnant and stale.

Personal hygiene is of utmost importance.

And think about this:

In the morning the kids head for school but before leaving the door they get the iodine spray in each nostril and the mouth. At the end of day when home from school the same thing is done. This is a very simple and effective measure to decrease viral load. And repeat it at bedtime.

In the evening ultraviolet irradiation can be given to the classroom.

Say there is a large public event at Madison Square Garden. Before the event each dog can be used to screen up to 700 people per hour. This can be used for people entering the event. After the event the dogs are used to help localize areas that need additional disinfection. Ultraviolet lights can be used here and even in the subway.

As far as restaurants ultraviolet irradiation at night and even using the dogs to help localize particular areas that need additional disinfection may be helpful.

Personal hygiene with facemasks, increased social distancing, and handwashing continue to be essential. Consider limiting public touch screens at information centers and museums.

This is a new American experience with social aspects of handling the pandemic. Many people want instant information and no errors. We are still learning, We need to obtain experience with this to handle any future pandemic in a safe manner. In my opinion, the above special measures may be effective.

We live in a world with viruses and we need to learn how to survive. Politicians started with a FEAR game. This may have been necessary to get Americans to accept wearing a mask and following other precautions. Now change that game plan using some common sense. Diminishing FEAR should include the press.

Most people can improve personal hygiene. Iodine spray is simple and inexpensive.

If you raise dogs this can be an initiative to modern treatment of a pandemic. Maybe the Westminster Annual Dog Show will have a Corona Specialist competition next year. Note I said next year. Patience, and this takes time— although many times I do not practice my own advice.

https://reason.com/2020/08/14/did-sweden-accidentally-blunder-into-covid-19-herd-immunity/

https://www.pix11.com/news/coronavirus/bronx-queens-showed-most-positives-on-antibody-tests

https://www.studyfinds.org/coronavirus-test-via-breathalyzer/

IV

Part Four

Actions, options, solutions, and procedures. Life is about survival, here is what you can do starting today to propel yourself in the right direction going forward. Continue to seek out the truth.

62

Monolaurin and
Hydroxychloroquine

SENT TO MY PATIENTS 8 AUGUST 2020:

There is a lot of concern regarding the recent coronavirus. Viruses are part of our world and will never be eliminated.

The best measures are personal hygiene as well as eating a wholesome diet.

No vaccination has been released at this point. One significant preventive measure is **monolaurin**. Coconut oil has lauric acid which our body converts into monolaurin. The importance of this is that monolaurin has a tremendous antiviral quality. I had one patient with HIV who had high viral loads. These dropped down considerably after using monolaurin and no other change in his treatment. I had the same happen in a patient who had chronic active hepatitis C. This covers all viruses.

So, monolaurin is not specific and it has a tremendous antiviral effect. Taking a scoop of this on a daily basis for maintenance is good. Symptoms suggestive of the flu increase to three or four times daily.

This is a natural and highly successful preventive measure.

I refer you to Healthnatura.com. They have an excellent product and one scoop or level teaspoon provides **3000** mg of the monolaurin. This is a good maintenance dose. If you look at other products you will see they are not quite this same concentration or dosage.

Hydroxychloroquine has been used for treatment of Corona. This is also been approved for prevention. In New York the drug is not available outside a hospital or without special permission.

I work with a pharmacy that can supply to patients in New York. A preventive dose is one tablet two times a week.

Let me know if you are interested in this option and how I can help. I am available to talk with you if you have questions regarding these preventive measures. Sometimes a patient does not need to be on both this and monolaurin at the same time.

I hope you get through the recent viral threat in good health.

CHRIS AND CORONA

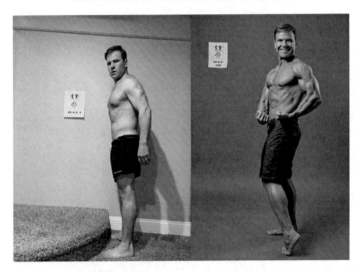

This is not an advertisement, and this is not me.

I have a young patient (pushing 50) who had a beneficial encounter with the coronavirus earlier this year.

I have worked with this patient for probably eight years. He is very disciplined, particularly in the last two years. He just could not get rid of that last belly fat.

One year ago, he weighed 172 pounds had a total body fat of 18.8%, with a 21% android distribution. An exam a year earlier his weight was the same with a total body fat of 17.8% and an android distribution of 24%. Comparison of exams showed that he had lost 2 # muscle and increased fat 1 #. He just maintained a little bit around the middle. His weight was stuck this year in January at 166 pounds. Then he went to 181 with corona.

Current weight is 159 pounds. For the past 90 days his diet has been macro with 40 g protein, 30 g carbs, 20 g of fat per meal 4 times a day. 130 ounces of water daily is taken.

The carbs were all complex consisting of sweet potatoes,

Ezekiel bread, rice, and oatmeal. Supplements and hormone optimization have been stable for years and not changed during this time. I hope this impresses the importance of the diet and how it is very frequently misunderstood. Fats don't make us fat. Carbohydrates do.

February, he started taking monolaurin at the onset but was sick with the virus for about a week. He said during that time he would just eat a few carbs that tasted good since he was not feeling well. If he was not able to take in some carbs at that time his body would have begun to break down muscle for calories. That is not good. The downside of not carrying too much fat is that there really is not much reserve for energy sources if there is no intake of calories.

I communicated with the patient as he began to get back into his exercise routine. He said he went to his prior diet that restricted carbs.

Not everyone is looking for on body habitus like this. The other thing is that many do not entirely understand what goes on with the physiology.

With the low-level activity during the day people will burn their own fat or any fat that is consumed. Eating fat does not make you fat. Patients state that they go through exercise and say they need their carbs for energy. Carbs are only needed for a short period of time during the exercise. They are not needed the rest of the 24-hour day. Most of the 24 hours a person is not burning calories like they were doing exercise. This is not a matter of so many calories in and so many calories out. Such a simple concept which is disregarded by the majority of practitioners and patients.

Chris achieved what he wanted. He lost 6 pounds (from January baseline) and is currently at 159 pounds.

Fat does not make you fat. Just make sure it is good fat and not canola oil. Carbs make you fat. Carbs are what keep the majority of Americans outside their optimal body composition. This comment is a very significant factor.

https://www.webmd.com/diet/ss/slideshow-belly-fat-facts?ecd=wnl_spr_080820&ctr=wnl-spr-080820_nsl-LeadModule_title&mb=lGVdiurmHBMQOzQukn1aapAy-WFWqf9PLEH%2foKnlpKv4%3d

https://www.linkedin.com/pulse/monolaurin-viral-infections-joseph-edward-bosiljevac-jr-md-phd-facs/?trackingId=RJGh%2BI-hZJVmJh3tJKHKDew%3D%3D

63

Liability Issues

I review many information sources and this is a professional memo for physicians. I also continue to communicate with patients.

There was a recent announcement of a bill signed by Gov. Cuomo. Whether this is right or wrong, I do not know. However a lot of changes are going on in society as a result of the pandemic, and New York is a state of high liability. You cannot belch on the sidewalk without a high liability of risk.

Restaurants need to take measures yet also worry about liability. What if someone accuses the restaurant as the source of a coronavirus infection.

Personal responsibility for hygiene and health are essential. Society needs to learn how to manage a pandemic. This can happen again.

5 AUGUST 2020: Medical Society of New York Article

<u>Cuomo Signs Bill to Roll Back Medical Liability</u>

Protections

Gov. Andrew Cuomo signed a bill that would reverse some of the medical liability protections provided to doctors, hospitals and nursing homes during the pandemic.

The bill was opposed by lobbying groups representing the health care industry as potentially adding to medical malpractice costs after workers risked their own health to treat COVID-19 patients. The law, which will be applied prospectively, reduces the level of legal immunity for doctors treating non–COVID-19 patients whose care is affected by the pandemic.

Hospitals and doctors had sought that cover as they were asked to take dramatic steps to respond to the pandemic, such as converting non-clinical spaces into treatment areas and asking doctors and nurses to work outside their specialty areas.

Statement of MSSNY President Dr. Bonnie Litvack, in Reaction to Governor Signing into Law Rolling Back COVID-19 Liability Protections

"We are deeply concerned with the consequences of the significant narrowing of these liability protections, particularly when there remains a very real possibility of a second surge of cases this fall. It will put our physicians and other health care workers, who not long ago were regularly lauded as 'heroes', into even more extraordinarily challenging circumstances. During the height of the pandemic, in many downstate hospitals, physicians and physicians in training were regularly being asked to provide health care services outside of their areas of expertise to help manage the overwhelming patient flow. They did so because of their dedication to helping their patients.

We pray that such a drastic situation will not come again, but if it does, many physicians will again find themselves with the unimaginable choices of triaging which patients are to receive care first, knowing full well that this new law means that the "wrong choice" could result in that physician losing everything they own to a lawsuit. Moreover, this narrowing of these liability protections also puts a physician at much greater risk of a lawsuit if the state once again requires the postponement of elective surgeries to preserve resources for patients with COVID-19. This is a grossly unfair position in which to be placed.

We are very concerned that the practical effect of this legislation will be that hospitals will face far more difficulties in attempting to manage a huge influx of patients in the event of a second surge.

To paraphrase David Bowie, apparently our doctors were heroes just for one day.

http://www.mssnyenews.org/covid-19/covid-19-update/

https://www.linkedin.com/pulse/apocalyptic-virus-joseph-edward-bosiljevac-jr-md-phd-facs/?trackingId=x930VCZ4Qq27T4n(

64

Physician Beliefs

MSSNY ENEWS: AUGUST 19, 2020 – NEARLY HALF OF PHYSICIANS BELIEVE COVID-19 WILL NOT BE UNDER CONTROL UNTIL AFTER JUNE 2021

The Physicians Foundation just released its biennial *Survey of America's Physicians,* revealing the impact of the COVID-19 pandemic on physician practices and their patients. The first part of the three-part series findings include:

§ The majority (86%) of physicians believe COVID-19 won't be under control until January 2021, with nearly half (49%) not seeing the virus being under control until after June 1, 2021.

§ A majority (72%) of physicians believe that the virus will severely impact patient health outcomes due to delayed routine care during the pandemic

§ 59% of physicians see opening businesses, schools and public places as a bigger risk to patients than continuing policies of isolation.

The other announcement on August 7 is that a green light

has been given to open all schools in the State of New York. There is still a lot of controversy about opening schools and restaurants. Teachers here in New York are talking about striking, but they still get their salary and pension. Restaurants are in a different game since overhead continues and there is no income. The FEAR factor is still in play.

https://www.linkedin.com/pulse/can-more-simple-joseph-edward-bosiljevac-jr-md-phd-facs/?published=t

http://www.mssnyenews.org/enews/august-19-2020/#covid

65

How do I feel? Coronavirus Pandemic

21 August 2020

There are no tourists. No hotels. No Broadway plays. New York has seen many small mom-and-pop businesses close for good. Restaurants and bars are open for outside service. There has been a benefit of free bus rides that have been provided since March but this will stop August 31. Gyms open September 2. Street traffic is about 60% normal.

New York one year ago was vibrant, fun, and active. August is always slow for New York City but this is worse and follows five months of shut down. This is super dead.

My practice is age management and for at least five months my office has been closed. I do not do any urgent care. It is beginning to pick up a little but many interested patients that live outside this state or this country are reluctant to come to New York at this time.

Every day I wake up and remember my grandmother told me "if you open your eyes it is already a good day." As far as work the door was slammed closed mid-March. I just finished a divorce in the New York system and basically my savings are gone. This has been a little hard for a guy pushing 70 years old. I feel the economic effect like many small businesses.

I have a brother from the Navy who served as a SEAL. His career has been one of survival and escape. So according to him, if I have my eyes open start from there.

So far I have survived. I like my work and feel that I can help people improve conditions that are not responsive with conventional medical care. I am healthy and I want to keep going. I will continue to work on my book and share my background and experience with patients so they can improve their health. I feel I am happier and healthier than 30 years ago.

1 September 2020

Today I received some help. The lease on my apartment runs out the end of the month. I talked to the manager and explained that my office had been closed for five months. I was asking for a little bit of a break. He told me if I would sign a year's lease at the same rate they would give me 2 month's rent free. Wow! I really appreciate this property management company because many landlords would not choose to do such. Even a small break on the rent for businesses as well as apartments shows that everyone is in this together and can help each other. Thank you, God.

There was an announcement on August 7 that a green light has been given to open all schools in the state of New York. There is still a lot of controversy about opening schools and restaurants. Teachers here in New York are talking about striking, but they continue to get their salary and pension. The FEAR factor is still in play. Many decision makers are not severely affected economically.

On September 1 the controversy about opening up schools was delayed, primarily by the teachers union and mayor De Blasio, but not teachers in general. Many teachers are anxious to do what is right for the children. They need to be in school. There are social aspects here. This not only gives them time to socialize and mature but also learn better hygiene as a normal routine.

We are still learning. I will continue to follow this pandemic. More common sense means this can be done more simply.

https://www.linkedin.com/pulse/can-more-simple-joseph-edward-bosiljevac-jr-md-phd-facs/?published=t

66

Look At These Numbers

2 September 2020

These comments come from an old man sitting on his porch. Actually I am on my fourth floor balcony in the Upper East Side New York City. I have a book to read in a moment, but I reviewed this electronic news statement from the Medical Society of New York.

2 SEPTEMBER 2020: MSSNY ENEWS

Siena Poll: New Yorkers Still Support Forced Closures

New Yorkers are still solidly in favor of shutting down large parts of society in an attempt to slow the spread of the coronavirus, according to a poll released by the Siena College Research Institute on Wednesday. A total of 70 percent of respondents say state government should prioritize the containment of the coronavirus, "even if it hurts the economy." Only 23 percent think the state should "restart the economy, even if it increases the risk to public health." That is basically the same result as when Siena asked the question in early July, when respondents favored public health 70-22.

"Don't Rush on Schools."

Pollsters also asked about several specific institutions and activities, and by and large, New Yorkers were not in a rush to have them return to normal. On public schools, only 18 percent said that they should reopen for all students immediately, while 33 percent said they should reopen with some sort of a hybrid model. A total of 46 percent said they should stay "closed for now and provide remote instruction as best as teachers can to all students."

Only 27 percent said that colleges "should bring students back to campus for the fall semester" while 66 percent said their courses should be entirely remote. Respondents were also asked about six different types of activities and whether they "now feel comfortable" participating in them:

- "Visiting a museum" was the only one that anything close to a majority — 45 percent, in this case — say they would be willing to do.
- A total of 38 percent said they are willing to dine indoors, though only 24 percent would be willing to drink at a bar.
- Thirty-one percent said they would be comfortable going bowling and 27 percent are OK going to the gym. And 23 percent would like to go to a movie theater, an activity that Cuomo still has not authorized.
- Siena also asked people how their behaviors have changed in recent months. Forty-two percent said

they have gained weight, 32 percent lost weight and 22 percent copped to consuming "more alcohol than usual." (Sept. 2 Politico NY Pro)

Look at these numbers. Many of the respondents state that the government should prioritize containment. Many people making decisions are minimally affected by the economic aspects. This is a virus. Viruses are part of our environment. Viruses will continue to be spread by people. There should be a balance of social and personal responsibility of the individual. We are learning. Fear still appears to be a big aspect with pandemic at this time.

Think about this— New York City has been kicked back because of the coronavirus. The incident before that was 9/11.

Let me take a step further. In the early 1970s I saw a movie with Jennifer O'Neill called *"Reincarnation of Peter Proud."* I have the book and it probably read it five or six times. After I read it again recently I started to look up other books by this author from Garden City, Long Island named Max Ehrlich. His first book (The Big Eye) relates to an empty New York City filled with fear. He describes New York City and Idlewild Airport during the Cold War about 1960. Much of this sounds similar to the current pandemic. Note: today Idlewild airport is named JFK.

I wanted to share a little bit of New York history coming from a Midwesterner living in Manhattan for 13 years and through the entire pandemic. Anyway, read a book by Max Ehrlich. Peter Proud is impressive.

https://www.linkedin.com/pulse/can-more-simple-joseph-edward-bosiljevac-jr-md-phd-facs/?published=t

http://www.mssnyenews.org/covid-19/mssny-enews-september-2-2020/#siena

67

Supercomputer Analysis of COVID-19

What happens if a supercomputer looks at the current coronavirus? I respect this kind of scientific work which explains more about the underlying biochemistry, physiology, and pattern of spread. We are still learning.

The ACE 2 receptors are important and a potential entry site for the coronavirus to enter and initiate an infection.

They may be regulated by medications, sex, and age which can all be variables as far as infection rate. Some medications can be used to inhibit this entry point. Looking at the physical structure of the coronavirus which shows multiple spikes on the surface.

These attach to the ACE 2 receptors. There is even a recent article talking about nanobodies that can cover up the spikes and prevent infection.

Inhibiting ACE receptors affects the renin-angiotensin system which control so many aspects of the circulatory system. Some of the COVID-19 symptoms may affect the heart or circulatory system through this mechanism.

The coronavirus can act as a natural ACE inhibitor, leading to cough and fatigue, gastrointestinal symptoms, and loss of taste and smell. CBD protects the ACE receptor so it will not accept a corona attack.

Buildup of a chemical called bradykinin certainly affects aspects of the infection including virulence and resultant symptoms. This also may be an aspect as far as the lung complications with coronavirus.

An interesting aspect is the suggestion that vitamin D is a potentially useful COVID-19 drug.

Recall that this is not really a vitamin but a hormone and most Americans are walking around with gutter levels of vitamin D in their system. The lower the vitamin D leads to an increase morbidity and mortality with the illness.

The researchers point out that the testing of any of these pharmaceutical interventions should be done in a well-designed clinical trial. Conventional medicine many times looks for a pill as a cure. If you believe in magic bullets then just close this book.

If the patient's underlying health is not good the body may not heal, recover, or respond to some medications. There is personal responsibility here.

The current approach with conventional medicine is to find a cure for what is going on. Our society is slow to accept personal hygiene items that protect society as a whole. Many say masks interfere with their personal rights.

The big argument now is how to contain the virus. There are many businesses here in Manhattan that are suffering. I have pointed out before that opening businesses and large public events can be more simple, but I am not a politician.

My approach today is to reboot cells. Yes there are other

biochemical mechanisms being understood. If I do the right thing for the body today it will heal itself.

Reboot cells to function more optimally. The body wants to heal itself.

https://www.linkedin.com/pulse/what-does-mean-reboot-joseph-edward-bosiljevac-jr-md-phd-facs/?trackingId=88mBPptfTYs CPcLZDIxQ%3D%3D

https://elemental.medium.com/a-supercomputer-analyzed-covid-19-and-an-interesting-new-theory-has-emerged-31cb8eba9d63

https://www.ibtimes.com/coronavirus-treatment-cannabis-enzymes-could-help-block-gateway-covid-19-study-2979422

https://phys.org/news/2020-09-nanobody-covid-infection.html

https://www.linkedin.com/pulse/cbd-corona-joseph-edward-bosiljevac-jr-md-phd-facs/?trackingId=KImoSlMcS8eU-qXEXUNBbjw%3D%3D

https://www.ibtimes.com/coronavirus-treatment-cannabis-enzymes-could-help-block-gateway-covid-19-study-2979422

68

Outrageous Myths of Coronavirus

The topic of this article (see link at end of chapter) interested me. My personal comments and opinions are presented as you read through the 13 items listed.

1. Viruses do not travel 5G but there is a possibility that 5G can cause viruses to mutate. The data is not complete here. There was data with 2G showing mutations of viruses. 3G and 4G have not been studied. Now let's do a mixture with an electronic environment of 2G through 5G. What can go on with that?

2. All of this really doesn't matter because an apocalyptic virus can come from some other source. We need to have personal health and develop social aspects for possible future infections. The testing itself is something new and we are learning from this as far as how to control the epidemic. In the meantime the politicians and press tend to generate anxiety and fear. Appropriate? I do not know, but that is where we are on September 4, 2020.

3. How bad is this virus? Or does this really emphasize poor underlying health including obesity? There are many subtle signs and people do not recognize that they are not healthy. The body cannot heal itself.

4. A current medical model predicts that 300,000 people may die from COVID-19 by December. It is essential for physical fitness to push the body to survive. Most Americans are not doing the basics to get better. So who is liable? Part of this is people don't not really understand true health. *"Viruses mutate all the time," says Jha, the Harvard doctor. "Most of them have no clinical biological significance," adding: "I haven't seen any data at least that I'm aware of that compels me to think that the virus has become any more or any less lethal."* There is a people problem—personal health.

5. Alcohol is a risk factor!! Meet me down at the bar. We need to talk about this.

6. So garlic is for vampires? It has a tremendous antiviral effect. There are many natural agents that can help fight infection. Monolaurin is one. Ingesting bleach makes no sense, except maybe when things are not presented well in the literature. Probably 50% of persons in this country are not truly healthy. People do not feel acutely ill but they are not healthy. When they get struck with something severe like the coronavirus it may result in very bad results.

7. I'm not going to comment much on hydroxychloroquine because we really need to talk about rebooting cells and personal maintenance and not a magic bullet. *I share office*

with a physician who has taken care Donald Trump in the past. The week when President Trump declared that he was taking a course of hydroxychloroquine, the office had so many calls from news agencies to find out if this particular doctor had prescribed the hydroxychloroquine!!!!

8. School kids need to wear a mask and do careful hand-washing. They can have their nose and mouth sprayed with an iodine spray before and after school. This is a very simple method that is tolerated very comfortably with no side effects. This kills virus. At night the school rooms can be irradiated with ultraviolet light to kill virus and other microbes. A social aspect also for the schools is promotion of personal hygiene. This is beneficial for societal gain.

9, 10, 11, 12. **Personal health is really a key. Less than 50% of Americans are _truly_ healthy.** The big deal are crowded rooms with poor ventilation. Masks show respect and can help decrease airborne spread of the virus. A scientific study is not needed as far as the ability of masks to prevent infection. Minimally, out of personal respect, masks should be used despite individual thoughts about restriction of personal freedom. This is a start to public acceptance of certain measures at times, such as during an epidemic. Clear plastic divisions set up in offices and restaurants or at the counter in retail stores may become routine.

13. As far as herd immunity, a lot of this may have to do with politics. Herd immunity was achieved in Sweden with very low fatality despite minimal closing for businesses and schools. Current antibody testing of patients in Queens

County, New York indicates that 58% of patients have antibodies. This should diminish the effects of a second outbreak this fall in this area.

Herd immunity is occurring slowly. This is a world where the viruses will continue to spread wherever there are humans. We need to learn how to do prevention in the safest manner possible. Personal hygiene, improved personal health, and isolation of high risk patients during epidemic are key items. Lifestyle aspects and physical fitness are essential. The only way we know more about pandemics is to do the extensive testing, evaluate, and learn. An apocalyptic virus may yet come, but businesses and schools may not have to be closed.

MYTHS OF EATING OUT

Yesterday after working at the desk for a while I went out for a two hour walk through Central Park. I did not feel like cooking so on my way back I stopped at a Thai restaurant and ordered a Pineapple Shrimp Medley to go.

The reason for this communication is to demonstrate subtle things regarding our lifestyle and diet that many times are not taken into account.

1. The pineapple came from a can so this was not fresh.
2. It contained small shrimp and I suspect that these were farm raised rather than wild.
3. The dinner was cooked in oil. If this was canola oil that is not healthy.
4. As far as a delivery I came home with the food encased

in plastic. I immediately emptied this out onto a plate and out of the plastic.

5. I minimize any use of the microwave because this may affect the structure of water in the food and make the food less nutritious.

So, on paper, this was a good meal. Sources of the food and cooking methods are gray areas which many people do not consider how they affect the nutrition of the food. The first step is to start thinking healthy. The second step is to start understanding what healthy really means.

https://elemental.medium.com/the-13-most-outrageous-covid-19-myths-and-misconceptions-14f4b532abbf

https://www.linkedin.com/pulse/dehydration-ii-joseph-edward-bosiljevac-jr-md-phd-facs/?trackingId=hp53qCu-jYnWwO5uRGl8XFQ%3D%3D

69

Common Sense and Corona

On **September 19, 2020** I took a flight out of LaGuardia to work one week in Ohio. First of all, Terminal One is finished and is very modern and up-to-date. Social distancing and wearing masks was enforced.

Now let me mention a little bit about common sense. I was carrying medical equipment so I had scheduled first class. Instead of allowing first class members to board, the airplane followed the procedure where the last rows filled first and slowly in sections the rest of the plane was filled. On disembarkation the airline crew requested that everyone remained seated except for the sections that were called to exit the plane.

My reaction? The plane filled very easily without people mulling all over each other and was completed in about one third of the time compared to what has been my usual experience over the years. This is such a common sense approach. Why it was never done before is probably related to America's lack of exposure to a pandemic.

In Ohio, restaurants were closed about three months

except for delivery. On this current trip the restaurants had been open for about three months. Social distancing was practiced inside as well as the employees wearing facemasks. They were serving about 75% capacity in the restaurants.

It has worked out in Ohio but the politicians are having a hard time using their common sense here in New York.

Let us take this a step further. Ultraviolet lights can be used to irradiate inside restaurants and classrooms during the night to kill virus. In addition iodine spray can be used to inhibit viral growth.

Over the past years approximately 100,000 people die annually with the influenza virus. Nothing major has been said about <u>victims</u> and <u>fear</u> with those statistics. Now the coronavirus is at fault (the news says it is Trump). Why all the sudden with this newest virus are those affected by it called 'victims'? It is word play that is giving the public a different feel about health. Personal health is still the same as it always has been, maybe this will help us take it more seriously. The anxiety of 2020 can subside when you take matters into your own hands.

The most important aspect is personal hygiene with masks and handwashing. Until now, American coronavirus prevention habits were not good.

Following other common sense such as the airline seating, ultraviolet lights in certain public areas, and the use of an iodine spray that can be given to children before and after school may definitely decrease the annual death rate from the H flu virus this year. If that is the case it will demonstrate that there will always be some "victims" of an epidemic / pandemic. However the mortality rate can be decreased by improving personal hygiene and using some of these other common sense answers.

Another point is the use of monolaurin, a coconut oil derivative that has a tremendous antiviral effect.

Finally, the highest mortality rate in all age groups are those patients that are not medically healthy but also have gutter levels of vitamin D. So significant.

How about dogs? I have mentioned the use of dogs to help locate virus clusters after large gatherings and events. Clusters could be left on surfaces, in bathrooms or anywhere that a large group of people left behind after and event. Once located by dogs the cluster can be neutralized and the space left safe for further use in the future.

Personal health maintenance is also important because today's lifestyle, including fast food and obesity, makes the risk of morbid complications higher. Personal hygiene and health requires some discipline. No, this is not against First Amendment rights. This is personal respect.

I suggest we follow some common sense rules as best we can. We cannot eliminate all mortality. If we see that the new coronavirus cases stay stable, even if they are not zero, and that H flu virus deaths decrease because of measures that have been implemented for coronavirus (with masks and handwashing), this would certainly support common sense effective actions for resistance and survival.

https://www.linkedin.com/pulse/corona-patient-how-difficult-diagnosis-bosiljevac-jr-md-phd-facs/?trackingId=d6xX%2Bu PEbaFaUYwaAA%3D%3D

https://www.linkedin.com/pulse/dogs-vs-corona-joseph-edward-bosiljevac-jr-md-phd-facs/?trackingId=uhHclVX6DVQiAr6JoMQaVw%3D%3D

70

Nitric Oxide Deficiency and Coronavirus

Here is an interesting article emphasizing the importance of nitric oxide. This was based on the COVID-19 epidemic. The mechanism affects the lining of the blood vessels and also the lung tissue that can be affected by coronavirus. I have talked previously about nitric oxide.

A point I would like to make is that nitric oxide is a basic part of normal healing. In many patients this is depleted which would definitely affect the response of that patient to an infection and also influence recovery. This is starting from behind in the ballgame to try to increase depleted levels.

Supplementation and diet can affect nitric oxide levels. In this study inorganic nitrogen in the diet was used to improve the formation of nitric oxide. For me the emphasis of this article is that nitric oxide is a basic part of our routine metabolism. Wound healing principles should be followed for positive effects.

Age management recommends correcting suboptimal

nitric oxide levels. Nitric oxide levels can be determined using a simple swab stick on an office visit. Although I feel this should be part of a routine physical, I will bet that 99% of patients have never had this done. My emphasis again goes to the use of wound healing principles with tissue repair, regeneration, and recovery.

I have seen many middle-age men with borderline high blood pressure that also had low nitric oxide levels. Nitric oxide relaxes blood vessels to dilate. When these levels were improved blood pressure drops down to the normal range. No meds needed.

I once had an 84-year-old gentleman who was taking Cialis and had an active sex life.

One day he came into my office and told me the Cialis was not working. Nitric oxide relaxes blood vessels and allows that guy below to get big and hard.

This encounter was years ago and I was just beginning to use the nitric oxide office test. I measured his nitric oxide levels and they were low. We started on a supplement for this and he started to include red beet powder with his protein shakes.

Three months later he comes back for a return visit. I asked him how his little guy was working. He told me he did not have to use the Cialis anymore.

Again, I comment—this is a basic part of wound healing and regeneration.

As I am writing up this article, a Han Solo movie is on TV. I remember his character as having a genuine manly love for the opposite sex. The thing that I catch is when he states "Women always get to know the truth."

https://www.sciencedirect.com/science/article/pii/S12864579203008

http://www2.cenegenics.com/e/49072/blog-saga-nitric-
oxide-/bswcsn/512904497

71

The Therapeutic Use of NAD

NAD (nicotinamide adenine dinucleotide) is an essential metabolite in our biologic system. It is found in cells in the mitochondria and as a coenzyme encourages ATP to produce energy (see diagram of Krebs cycle). With sufficient energy the cell functions optimally. A cell producing suboptimal energy leads to degenerative conditions and even cancer. NAD is used in every cell in the body that has mitochondria. NAD treatment was first used clinically in patients with chronic alcoholism and drug addiction. A course of intravenous therapy can markedly decrease or eliminate cravings.

After age 50 it has been demonstrated that NAD levels continue to decrease significantly in most of us. This leads to fatigue because cell energy production is diminished. Many of the CEOs I treat that entertain nightly have depleted even more NAD with alcohol consumption. The most impressive finding for me is the fact that patients with chronic neurodegenerative conditions such as multiple sclerosis have nerve cells that have dumped out all their

NAD, which then presents as abnormal nerve function, neuropathies, and pain.

NAD can be given in many forms. By mouth it has to be a component of nicotinic acid. Pushing this at high levels causes hot flashes and other symptoms that patients do not like. Oral niacinamide and resveratrol can help improve NAD levels but this may take 90 days or more. This is why an intravenous infusion is a good start. Patches and creams can be used or even a nasal spray. Liposomal NAD is now also available.

My preference is giving an intravenous infusion as a bolus. With this route we know the medication is getting directly into the bloodstream. Following that we can help support NAD levels with oral supplementation.

The infusion itself takes in the range of about four hours and can be performed in an office or at a patient's home. Preferential treatment would be an initial IV of a Myers cocktail (B vitamins and Vitamin C), methyl cobalamin (B12) and glutathione. Once this is infused then anywhere from 500 to 1000 milligrams of NAD can be administered intravenously.

NAD encourages biologic activities that involve methylation. This is a word referring to how the body is metabolizing substances. Trimethyl glycine (betaine) provides a good methyl donor and can be taken as an oral supplement. This is a good methylator which can lower homocysteine (inflammation) levels. Otherwise, additional oral magnesium, calcium, and potassium are helpful. Hydrogen water may hydrate the cell to work better (subsequent article)— see how it is involved with the NAD process in the diagram.

Figure 6.11A An overview of the Krebs cycle

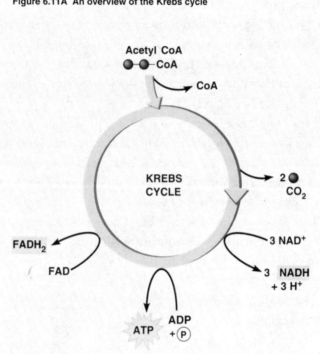

As far as the infusion, the IV needs to be administered at a rate that takes about four hours since faster infusion can bring on uncomfortable but not life-threatening side effects such as dizziness and chest tightness. These are eliminated by controlling the rate of infusion and is related to the assimilation of the NAD into the cell. Occurrence varies depending on the patient. It is interesting that alcoholics will rapidly soak up lots of NAD with no adverse side effects. They are severely depleted. The liver is an organ that requires a lot of NAD.

I have had patients who showed remarkable short-term improvement in neurologic dysfunction following intravenous NAD infusions. Any symptoms to the NAD infusion are temporary (this is a normal biologic product)—you are filling up the NAD gas tank.

One example is a 55-year-old patient with MS who came to me in a wheelchair. He had not been able to walk for two months. Following the first intravenous NAD treatment the patient walked from his wheelchair into the bathroom on his own. There was also considerable improvement in his speech.

NAD alone can be used for many chronic neurodegenerative conditions. In **combination with stem cells I have seen** further improvement with:

1. Multiple Sclerosis
2. Parkinson's disease
3. Alzheimer's
4. Post stroke
5. Traumatic brain injury
6. Chronic degenerative neuromuscular diseases
7. Peripheral neuropathy

NAD can be **combined with stem cells** for rejuvenation.

A doctor and IV team needs to be certified to prescribe and administer NAD for medical treatment. Not every doctor can administer NAD and it is not available in most hospitals.

72

STEM CELL THERAPY: Stem Cells in Treatment of COVID-19 Cases - This is Wound Healing

On May 5, 2020 it was announced that three critically ill COVID-19 patients at Baptist Hospital in Miami were the first in the US to be successfully treated with stem cells. These patients had severe lung and respiratory complications of the illness. Within days the mesenchymal stem cells doubled oxygen levels in these patients.

On August 14, 2020 the University of Minnesota launched a stem cell trial to improve pulmonary signs and symptoms with severe COVID-19 patients.

On August 20, 2020 scientists at UCLA related their advances in using stem cells to take on COVID-19. This even includes an attempt to create an off-the-shelf cell therapy.

These are some national cases. There have been many more reports worldwide. Multiple groups have also shown similar results the past 5 years using stem cells with lung problems.

Consider the anatomy and physiology of these treatments. An intravenous injection goes to the right side of the heart which pumps blood into the lungs. Stem cells injected intravenously will be trapped in the alveolar capillary membrane and initiate their repair of the lung from that area. Recall that I previously indicated pneumonia and lung complications as the main cause of death with coronavirus. *Stem cells administered to a patient very ill with the coronavirus could help the pulmonary status.*

The first case reported was a 65-year-old female from Kunming, China treated with umbilical cord stem cells resulting in a remarkable recovery in two days.

Dr. Zhao from Shanghai University presented a small study including seven patients with favorable results using stem cells.

I found out at the **tail end of March** that a biotech company from Cleveland received permission from the FDA to treat coronavirus patients with severe lung complications and pneumonia using stem cells. I have been using stem cells for lungs with excellent results for five years. This makes me smile. Things are catching on for medical treatment.

Pneumonia and pulmonary dysfunction are the most frequent causes of death from the coronavirus. Patients with asthma, cigarette smokers, or those that have underlying heart disease are more susceptible to severe and fatal complications.

As a physician my initial objective is do no harm. The second is listen to the patient, observe, and examine. This is how I develop judgment and experience.

Ozone therapy has also been to improve oxygenation of severely ill COVID-19 patients. Ozone is improving oxygenation at the cellular level while cells are being rebooted in this example.

When I have used intravenous ozone it results in a 2 to 3% increase in oxygen saturation 30 to 45 minutes after the infusion.

Ozone is a highly energized form of oxygen found in nature. It consists of three oxygen atoms bonded together where oxygen primarily exists as two atoms. Ozone presents as a molecule with a third oxygen atom that is highly reactive and wants to leave the group. This provides the oxidant quality of ozone that can be used for our own health benefits. An oxidizer (oxidant) is different from a free radical. Oxidizers are not bad - they help us get rid of the "junk" that resides in our bodies. Ozone already has many industrial applications because of this characteristic. Dave Asprey explains the health benefits of ozone.

The First Patient

A 49-year-old man who had already required ICU admission was deteriorating on the ward. He had deteriorated to the point that he required oxygen at the highest concentration and yet it was oxygenating his lungs poorly. Intubation and connection to a ventilator was planned, but surprisingly, after the first session of Ozone therapy, the improvement was significant and oxygen requirements could be decreased.

Dr. Alberto Hernández explained that:

"The improvement after the first session of Ozone treatment was spectacular. We were surprised, his respiratory rate normalized, his oxygen levels increased, and we were able to stop supplying him with as much oxygen since the patient was able to

oxygenate himself.

To our surprise, when we carried out an analytical control, we observed how Ferritin, an analysis determination that is being used as a prognostic marker in this disease, not only had not followed the upward trend, but had decreased significantly; that decline continued in the following days. This result encouraged us to administer it to other patients who are following the same improvement as our first patient."

Ferritin (a blood test) was mentioned above, and this is part of my routine blood work when monitoring patients. It is an excellent marker for inflammation when elevated. It also correlates with recovery from the disease or condition when it decreases. That is a nice fact to know as additional data to help manage someone that is severely ill such as with the coronavirus.

This is an objective sign that can be used to follow the patient's progress.

This pandemic - and I live in the epicenter in Manhattan - allows an opportunity to see and feel the experience of this illness. What I publish about the coronavirus epidemic here in NYC is already past time. The ballgame continues to be played with further decisions pending. This may open up "out of the box" and untraditional lines-of-thinking for many people as far as treatment options.

Stem Cell Treatment

I am currently certified internationally to perform stem cell therapies. My practice is different and more diverse than most stem cell clinics. Overall I have treated more than 1000 cases of various sorts with stem cell therapy, mostly joint and soft tissue injections. Over 200 of all cases were with systemic treatment with IV administration.

This is all about wound healing—boost the healing potential of the body. I do not have a set recipe but use principles of wound healing learned as a surgeon. The patient is thoroughly evaluated using the human machine concept. Chemical and hormone balance is promoted to improve healing and regeneration. The condition to be treated is evaluated to determine how the stem cells will be administered—either a local injection or IV administration. An overall treatment program is developed using adjunctive services such as red light therapy and hyperoxygenation to promote healing and recovery. Reversing the inflammation from an autoimmune process is frequently a part of the program.

Background

I received a medical degree in 1975. My conventional training then consisted of a rotating internship and six years of surgical training. I became board-certified and had a solo cardiovascular surgery practice for 29 years near Kansas City. I became frustrated during my surgical career because patients were sent to me for surgery and they were on 20 different medicines. I saw positive results from chiropractic and other alternative treatments. This did not make sense from my conventional medical education.

At that point I obtained a doctorate in Natural Medicine and practiced some alternative methods along with cardiovascular surgery for several years. Now they can call me doctor/doctor.

My surgical career has provided a widespread background. I trained in the mid-1970s when there was not a lot of bureaucratic paperwork and rules to keep training physicians from performing procedures or learning to make treatment decisions. We learn from training and experience.

Furthermore, I spent a year at Charity Hospital in New Orleans to learn during a rotating internship at a large, general municipal hospital. My surgical residency lasted five years where experience and training was gained in multiple areas. I have seen and treated many patients the past 45 years. Good judgment comes from experience.

Balance

After my solo practice with cardiovascular surgery and alternate methods, I now practice the concept of practicing medicine using conventional American as well as alternative methods. I don't do surgery any more. I quit before I was told I was "getting a little slow."

The concept that the patient is a human machine and the entire organism needs to be addressed as part of the healing process is essential. This is all about wound healing.

At the age of 58 I received an offer to open an age management practice in New York City. I was single. All my kids are grown. This started a new adventure in my life. I closed the surgical practice in Kansas and have lived in Manhattan (not the Little Apple in Kansas) for 13 years.

Widespread experience

1. I trained before hospitalists (physicians working hourly

shifts taking care of hospital patients) so I was responsible for the workup of the patient, to learn to perform the surgical procedure, and total postoperative care of the patient.

2. As part of my background and training, I have operated or assisted with surgery on almost every body part. I have broad experience in conventional medicine and add "the other side of the fence" with natural medicine.

3. I have performed a dozen medical missions to Third World countries which include Bolivia, Honduras, Mexico, Colombia, and Dominican Republic. I speak Spanish very well so this is why I chose Latin third world countries. However, to see how these people handle their health was important to help me develop my current opinion of true health. Learning about healthcare in these areas and what these patients have used locally for health benefit significantly improved my thought process and practice.

Age Management

The main principle with age management is developing optimal chemical and hormone balance. The human machine needs to be balanced to optimize the ability to repair and heal. This balance supports wound healing that can improve results of stem cell procedures. Use of aspects from conventional medicine as well as natural medicine to approach this balance has been very successful. We are looking at complete, comprehensive treatment beginning with data collection during the initial workup that develops a good baseline to give direction. This provides a roadmap.

With an Age-Management practice, I quickly found that many patients have body parts that wear out. My experience with stem cells started with joint and soft tissue injections and includes treating retired NFL and NBA players as well as military special operations patients.

Prolozone injections for joints and soft-tissue problems has been used in my practice for many years. Sugar water and ozone as injections stimulate healing.

I have 13 years experience following and performing stem cell treatments. This started with extracting fat or bone marrow as the stem cell source, PRP (platelet rich plasma), and placental stem cell products. The last five years I have primarily used umbilical cord stem cells in my therapies. Part of the experience gained over the last 13 years is recognizing many times that after age 35 I may not want to use your own stem cells. They have been exposed to toxins in the environment and from your lifestyle for as many years as you are old.

This is even more so if the patient has a chronic, degenerative condition. The human machine needs to be balanced to optimize the ability to repair and heal. This is something that can improve results of stem cell procedures. Use of aspects from conventional medicine as well as natural medicine to approach this balance has been very successful. We are looking at complete, comprehensive treatment beginning with data collection during the initial workup that develops a good baseline to give direction.

I initially took care of professional service members of the military with bone and joint injuries. At the prompting by some of the officers I became involved with systemic conditions including traumatic brain injury with reasonable recovery.

I saw some systemic conditions, particularly those involved with chronic inflammation, can also improve. An example is ulcerative colitis. Additional adjunctive medications can be used here to affect inflammation so that the stem cell therapy is more effective.

Many other areas, such as central nervous system problems, can also be treated. There is an old time injection procedure performed commonly in the 1930s that was quite successful in its time for dealing with head and neck pain problems. This was the SPG block done by injection into the temporal area of the scalp. This was used to break a vicious cycle of migraine headaches.

Along comes the pharmaceutical industry about 1940 and the course of medicine encouraged patients to take a few pills instead of a shot. This injection technique became forgotten in conventional medicine, but not to this old-time surgeon. This technique is not taught in ENT programs today. To see improvement in central nervous system conditions is impressive, because this injection site allows entrance of stem cells into the head. I have seen traumatic scarring and MS lesions resolve after treatment. This also helps to balance the autonomic nervous system when the sympathetic aspect is dominant, such as conditions with chronic pain.

General Principles

As a physician, the first principle with stem cell treatment is: **DO NO HARM**.

To begin, I do not prefer your stem cells if you are over the age of 35 or younger if there is an autoimmune or chronic degenerative condition. They have been exposed to the environment as many years as you are old.

Umbilical cord stem cells are immune privileged. There are no tissue reactions or cancer risk when infused. I have never seen any adverse reaction to stem cell treatment.

So the primary risk of stem cell treatment is a needle stick into a joint or an intravenous infusion.

Some stem cell treatments can be done in one session but others may consist of several appointments over 4-6 weeks as part of the overall process. The clinical course is one of wound healing. The cells are rebooted to function more normally. A clinical assessment was performed and the game plan outlined from there.

Subsequent treatment may not consist of further stem cell infusion but will use adjuvant processes to improve overall wound healing.

Stem cell therapies are legal and medically accepted but currently exist outside of the insurance industry. In my experience, many times results are much better than with conventional treatment. This is about quality of life.

Adjuvant Therapies

Another important point is **biophysics**. Here electrical, light, magnetic, and other energy waves, and also some other defined or undefined sources are encountered. These energy sources can alter and enhance cell function and physiology.

One of the aspects to look at with stem cell treatment is wound healing. What can be done as an adjuvant treatment to promote and stimulate stem cell growth? These will be covered in detail in subsequent articles. One of the first aspects is establishing chemical and hormone balance as part of the age management and healing process. The next steps are:

1. Light therapy, oxygen, and certain biologic substances such as NAD (nicotinamide adenine dinucleotide) are essential adjuvants of the healing process. I rarely see these components provided in U.S. practice. The use of these modalities require certification and training not provided in medical education in this country. Light therapy uses a wavelength of light that stimulates nitric oxide production and stem cell assisted healing activity. Repeated post injection treatments can also be helpful. Results depend on administration using certain frequencies for delivery of the light, location of administration, and serial exams. Here we find light directing healing and repair.

2. Oxygen is administered using ozone in a manner that rivals hyperbaric oxygen treatment.

3. NAD infusions are essential in relieving neurologic symptoms in patients that have a chronic neurodegenerative condition such as multiple sclerosis. NAD infusions are not available in most offices including hospitals.

4. Exosomes can be administered in follow-up and serve as growth factors to stimulate stem cell activity.

5. Small proteins or peptides with specific biologic activity can be given as part of the course of wound healing.

6. What is the significance of the electromagnetic effects on cell function? Evidence on the 2G electromagnetic wave demonstrated that this can mutate viruses. No

further studies have been done on 3G or 4G. Now we have 5G. Not only that but you have a mixture in the environment of 2G through 5G. Here is a gray area. This potentially could be the source of an apocalyptic virus. What we learn as a society in maintaining the current pandemic can help in the future.

7. Pulsed electrical frequency therapy (PEFT) is another type of bioenergy that can be used to inhibit cancer cell growth.

So in summary:

- **Prepare the patient. Define the final goal and the plan to achieve this. It is more than just injecting stem cells to get an optimum result.**
- **Systemic optimization prior to the procedure will support stem cell results.**
- **Look at the injection procedure, which includes site injected, associated medications, and other aspects such as biophysics that can be used to support the stem cell therapy.**
- **Follow-up care subsequent to the injection is also an important part of recovery. An example is further red light laser therapy, again using various frequencies and location can help achieve optimum results.**

My position has allowed me as a clinical scientist to use observation and experience to help direct stem cell therapies. I look at things from an overall aspect— you are a Human Machine. That is part of being Dr./Dr.

Balance—the body wants to heal itself.

We continue to learn about the use of stem cells in the treatment of COVID-19 complications. This is an advance in medical knowledge. Prevention is most important. Stem cells and immune plasma provide treatment modalities that can help with severe symptoms.

I have a small private practice in NYC and am not involved with any institution or insurance program. I have had experience with stem cell treatments for 13 years. The majority of the treatments were for joint and soft tissue problems. The military has provided me with experience treating systemic conditions. These include include MS, strokes, emphysema, and cirrhosis. The results with emphysema and MS are good. <u>Wound healing principles and adjunctive measures that promote healing and recovery are essential for an optimal treatment program</u>. Keep this in mind when evaluating stem cell therapies for you or the family.

https://www.newsmax.com/health/health-news/stem-cell-research-biotechnology-umbilical-cord/2020/05/05/id/966202/

https://www.msn.com/en-us/health/medical/university-of-minnesota-launches-stem-cell-trial-against-severe-covid-19/ar-BB17XsJl

https://newsroom.ucla.edu/releases/stem-cell-research-covid-19

https://www.ncbi.nlm.nih.gov/pmc/arcles/PMC6739436/

www.mystemcelltherapy.com/2020/03/coronavirus-crically-
ill-chinese-paent-saved-by-stem-cell-therapy-study-says/

73

Are Stem Cell Therapies Warranted? This is Wound Healing

- There is always controversy about supervision and monitoring any new treatment in medicine.
- My opinions are presented after 13 years experience using stem cell therapies.
- The risk of harm is essentially zero depending on the experience of the practitioner
- Ripoff?— not in my practice and experience.
- Benefits— joint and soft tissue repair and treatment of some systemic conditions
- Systemic conditions I have treated include MS, other autoimmune conditions, emphysema, heart failure, cirrhosis, stroke, and traumatic brain injury.
- Repair—regeneration—rejuvenation— longer telomeres—younger system.

There is information in the recent news regarding stem cell

clinics that promise unapproved treatments.

What does this mean? There has to be supervision over medical products provided. The FDA uses regulation 361 HCT/P to monitor stem cells, and this looks at preparation of the product itself. The umbilical cord stem cells that I use have minimal manipulation other than cryofreezing and the addition of a microscopic amount of a sulfa agent as a stabilizer for storage.

Many clinical studies will be foreign-based. These studies are not easily approved by the FDA, even though these studies represent significant overall clinical experience.

The public assumes that the FDA has to approve specific medical therapies provided by a qualified professional to improve a patient's health. Stem cell therapies are not illegal. The FDA cannot interfere with a doctor-patient relationship. The real controversy may actually be focusing on this therapy to make money.

I trained in cardiovascular surgery via conventional medicine. I also have a second doctorate in natural medicine to provide a wide background and experience practicing medicine for 45 years.

After 29 years in a solo practice near Kansas City I moved to New York City and have been doing stem cell treatments for the last 13 years.

It is important for the patient to understand medical facts at layperson levels. This information can then be used to make an appropriate health decision. The concepts presented for the patient about stem cell therapy in this article:

1. **Harmful / Risk**

  2. **Ripoff**
  3. **What is the benefit?**

RISK

As a physician it is important for me to first **DO NO HARM**. With stem cells there is no tissue reaction. Umbilical cord stem cells are immune privileged. There is no cancer danger. So the big risk is a needlestick into a joint or an intravenous infusion.

My stem cell experience began with retired NFL and NBA players. Then came military special operations members (age 55 who continue to go on deployment and serve this country). The stem cell experience started with joint and soft tissue treatments initially, but with the military patients I have the opportunity to treat numerous cases of systemic disease. The list includes MS, other autoimmune conditions, traumatic brain injury, stroke, emphysema and lung problems, cirrhosis of the liver, ED, and even cases with cancer. Many of these resolved or improved significantly following wound healing and stem cell treatment.

If you were my brother with a medical condition that may benefit appropriately from stem cell treatment then I would not hesitate to give you a stem cell injection. However, for my brother I would use a big needle!

RIPOFF

In my 13 year experience with stem cell therapies I have extracted abdominal fat and bone marrow to obtain stem cells, used placental or amniotic fluid components, and now currently use umbilical cord stem cells. I have seen various companies come and go. It is important to review the scientific background and biologic information provided about the product and preparation.

Currently I use a company that delivers a cryofreeze specimen of umbilical cord stem cells and exosomes. The product comes from a group of women that are 18 to 35 years of age, medically screened upside down and inside out, and they go on and have a scheduled C-section. She gets the baby and the stem cell company gets the umbilical cord.

These specimens are preserved with <u>minimal manipulation</u> and cryofreezed. When thawed the specimen has been clinically evaluated so that it consistently has more than 90% active nucleated cells. Approximately 3 to 5% of these will be stem cells. The specimen also undergoes evaluation to see if certain growth factors are present to encourage healing. All of this meets FDA guidelines for delivering a product.

However, preparation and handling of the specimen may affect the number of active cells. Therapeutic handling is essential as far as wound healing and the use of stem cells in treatment.

From my experience, I will not use "stem cells" from" old people." 35-year-old stem cells have been exposed to a lot in our environment.

The stem cells provided are multipotent mesenchymal stromal cells. For the layperson these are called MSC. The cells divide, grow, and differentiate in about 90 days to a certain cell that can form cartilage, muscle, ligament, or perhaps improve the function of an internal organ. Clinical quantification of certain biologic activities is performed to be sure that the cells have the potential to differentiate and can serve for the clinical condition.

1. I trained as a cardiovascular surgeon through conventional medicine and also have a doctorate in natural medicine. I am certified in age management. I have international stem cell certification and certification for intravenous NAD administration. My background and experience is broad and extensive. At almost 70 years of age I have developed reasonably good judgment with a variety of stem cell cases.

2. My gray hair has gone away for whatever that is worth. Not my hair!!! It got thicker. Just the gray.

3. Stem cell therapies are <u>not</u> a **ripoff**. As a clinical scientist my observation and experience has demonstrated improvement in the majority of patients with stem cell treatments if done using proper wound healing principles.

4. There are adjunctive procedures available that improve overall results. With my surgical background I approach this using wound care principles. The use of light, oxygen, NAD, exosomes (which contain growth factors, a lot of micro RNA, and other bio proteins to stimulate various biological functions), and other methods which enhance wound healing and stem cell activity have significantly improved my results.

5. *This will be the future of medicine 20 years from now.*

6. Unfortunately there is politics and ignorance. Eighty percent of my medical colleagues and 80% of patients just do not get it. Many patients do not want to set up an acceptable discipline in their lifestyle to improve

their health. And there is always a cost to the patient if the procedure is not insurance approved.

7. Stem cells can provide repair, regeneration of tissue, and rejuvenation based on the ability to heal and appropriate discipline in lifestyle.

BENEFITS

Here is a patient example:

An 83-year-old white female with a 41 year history of MS came to see me about stem cell treatment. The patient was using a walker. She was falling frequently but had not broken anything yet. The patient had severe painful neuropathies in both legs and was controlling this with 8 pain pills a day.

I went through a full initial evaluation and began to use testosterone cream with her and some physical therapy. This increased leg muscle strength enough that she came into my office about six weeks later without the walker. She was now in a better mode for recovery.

To initiate the treatment with stem cells for a patient with a chronic neurodegenerative process, NAD is administered.

To review, in middle school we learned about the Krebs cycle. This is the cell's method to produce energy to function. NAD (nicotinamide adenine dinucleotide) is a coenzyme which is essential to assist the cell to produce normal energy. Cells producing normal energy function normally. With decreased energy production, a chronic or degenerative condition may develop, and maybe even cancer.

NAD levels go down as we get older. After age 50 it has significantly decreased. CEOs in my practice that entertain frequently with alcohol use may have lower levels yet. *Patients with chronic neurodegenerative disease have a condition where nerve cells will dump out their NAD. Then the neuropathies and all kinds of neurologic symptoms develop.*

In my experience, stem cell infusion has assisted many patients with MS as well as other autoimmune conditions. Because they all have low NAD levels, an infusion of 1000 milligrams of NAD is given intravenously for two days prior to the stem cells. With the NAD infusions I have noted immediate improvement in neurologic symptoms in many patients. The patient described stated that the painful neuropathy improved significantly for a few days. She also had a short time improvement in muscle strength and balance when she walked. This is all with the NAD infusion. Remember, this is just temporary since we are filling up their NAD gas tank. Oral supplementation has to be specific to increase NAD level significantly. The oral route also takes many months so the intravenous infusion is a nice bonus for most patients.

Many patients continue to improve after the stem cell infusion. In this particular patient after one month she had to take **ZERO pain pills**. She was walking with a cane. She was driving a car. She was more independent.

What is common is to see a slight relapse in symptoms around three months. This is at the tail end of the stem cell growth and differentiation process. Increased symptoms represent nerve cells regenerating. Another stem cell infusion is not necessary. At this point administration of exosomes (which contain many growth factor proteins and micro RNA) encourages further stem cell activity, wound healing, and continued improvement. *The symptoms go away because of the anti-inflammatory property of the stem cells and exosomes. I have seen this pattern in many patients.*

As a clinical scientist, observation and experience directs what is right for the patient.

I understand the societal concern because the system is not set up for insurance approval and payment. I gave up dealing with any insurance company 15 years ago. There is no third-party interfering with my judgment to do what is right for the patient.

Hopefully the information presented is helpful to review topics for discussion with your doctor regarding stem cell therapy.

As far as benefit:

1. Continued opportunity for qualified professionals to provide medical treatment with stem cell therapy will lead to reliable therapy.
2. The first objective is assurance for minimal risk to the patient.
3. The main goal of treatment is to improve quality of life.
4. I have a small practice in Manhattan with patients who trust me. This is rewarding and I have seen many patients get better.
5. This is an old man's opinion on stem cell therapy—In 20 years this will be state-of-the-art.
6. Then we go from there—exciting!!

https://www.nbcnews.com/health/health-news/many-stem-cell-clinics-promise-unapproved-treatments-how-stay-safe-n1072001

https://www.aaos.org/AAOSNow/2018/May/Research/research02/?ssopc=1

https://medicine.wustl.edu/news/surprising-culprit-nerve-cell-damage-identified/

74

STEM CELL THERAPY: My Experience for OPTIMAL RESULTS using *WOUND HEALING*

- Just injecting stem cells is not a complete procedure.
- Stem cell availability has increased with placental and umbilical cord blood sources.
- Proper chemical and hormone balance can get things on the right track for healing. When balance is not optimal, it is not worthwhile to go into the doctor's office, receive a shoulder injection, and expect miracles.
- Patients do not come to my office and just get an injection. They get balanced for healing.
- This is a process of wound healing.
- The location of the injection, the solution to be injected, and what additional agents that can be

included with the stem cells during the procedure and recovery also play a major part.
- **Good judgment comes from experience.**

One area of antiaging has to do with body parts that wear out. This happens from injury, athletics, and daily wear and tear. Joints can be repaired or replaced. One of the repairs may be stem cells.

My career change and move to New York City has led to significant experience in the field of stem cells. This started over 13 years ago with some retired NFL and NBA players. These players were going to Denver for stem cell injections of joints. The doctor there asked me to do prolotherapy injections on each patient several times to get the environment of the joint ready for healing prior to their stem cell injection. So I'm sitting there in front of a 320 pound former defensive player thinking about that involuntary knee reflex before administering the injection. Occasionally there can be violence in my profession.

First, to harvest stem cells there is a separate procedure where bone marrow is drawn from the hip bone. To process and concentrate the stem cells takes several hours. The specimen can then be injected later the same day back into the patient. Because of FDA regulations, stem cells cultured from the sample are considered a processed or manufactured medication which has not been authorized for use in the USA. Patients will travel to the Caribbean or other countries to receive these cultured cells by injection, which provides a higher concentration of stem cells. Are there differences in results with groups receiving cultured or non-cultured stem cells? Is there a minimal number of stem cells that correlate with the level of the result? This may be more directly related to other variables associated with wound healing than the stem cell infusion.

Another source of stem cells is adipose tissue which also requires a separate procedure to liposuction the fat as the source of the tissue.

Amniotic fluid and umbilical cord stem cells then became available. These sources are harvested from patients scheduled for a C-section. Donors are 18 to 35 years old and undergo extreme medical clearance. The fluid is obtained at the time of the C-section. These little cells are pluripotential— in other words, they can develop into anything. This has been shown with clinical experience.

One of the benefits is to save the patient an additional procedure for harvesting stem cells. The other thing to consider is what is the condition of stem cells that come from someone who is medically not very healthy? And older? Here the umbilical cord is a better source.

The stem cells have been filtered so there is no HLA, which is a protein that can cause an incompatibility reaction. Amniotic fluid and umbilical cord stem cells can be used universally and saves the patient from having a painful second procedure for harvesting.

Speaking with colleagues across the country about their experience with one type of case or another, these cells cannot and have not caused any allergic or incompatibility reaction over the years. So, very safe with good results.

Also, the list of medical conditions being treated seems unlimited. This is wound healing. The body wants to heal itself.

Now some important observations:

First, some of the retired professional players did better than others. This correlated closely with chemical and hormone balance of the human machine. Some were in metabolic shape where the body was not ready to heal anything. Patients in a degenerative, aging process and poor overall metabolic health may not have optimum results. Besides slow deterioration, chronic inflammation may not cause any acute pain or symptoms.

These guys were giving their own stem cells from hip bone marrow. How good are these cells that have been affected by environmental toxins for the same number of years as the patient's age? Stem cell source is important and availability of amniotic and umbilical cord stem cells can provide advantages.

Second, consider where to inject. Intra-articular and soft-tissue results are straightforward. It is useful for injecting Achilles and large tendon tears to prevent rupture and can be used to repair partial tendon ruptures, even inside the shoulder or other joint.

Injections for different types of facial pain and migraine headaches have greater than 70% success rate for long-term good relief and over 90% with some definite benefit. The injection for these is in the temporal area of the skull and is known as an SPG block (sphenopalatine ganglion).

Injections can be given for systemic conditions. Lung conditions are ideal since the first passage of the blood from an intravenous injection is into the lung. Every case of MS I have treated responded favorably. Ulcerative colitis and Crohn's disease have shown improvement.

Third, what else can be administered along with the stem cells? For instance, hyaluronic acid promotes restructuring of nervous tissue, particularly the nerve sheath or the insulation covering the nerve. This can be used when dealing with chronic nerve pain. Mixing stem cells with hyaluronic acid can help lengthen the duration of dermal fillers. And this is all natural tissue. Intra-articular injection of growth hormone also helps with cartilage formation.

This is not **just inject stem cells and all is good**. Here is my approach about stem cell treatment:

1. What is the goal or attempt to heal or repair? Judgment needs to be used because sometimes the injury is such that a surgical procedure is necessary. An injection alone would not be sufficient. However, an adjunctive stem cell injection can be considered to improve healing when surgical repair is performed.
2. As a surgeon with an over 40 year experience operating on many parts of the body, my widespread background and experience in both sides of medicine offers additional benefit. Look at dealing with an entire human machine.
3. It is important for chemical and hormone balance in the patient for proper healing. There is no current textbook or studies with proven recipes for stem cell administration. Judgment and experience is necessary. This is wound healing.
4. Look at the overall chemical and hormone balance of the patient. Borderline diabetic or elevated ferritin (indicating liver inflammation) levels can certainly affect results. This is like being a coach, training

patients and getting the human machine ready for healing. Sometimes a short adjunctive recovery course of growth hormone can get things started off well.

5. Where is the injection located? Looking at a goal long-term and possibly permanent healing, **location** can be very important as far as the result. Intra-articular and soft-tissue sources are easy enough. A sphenopalatine ganglion (SPG) block in the head can be very useful as a location to inject in the relief of many painful facial symptoms. Pain specialists frequently perform sympathetic denervation (disconnection) on the stellate ganglion to try to affect the overall autonomic nervous system. Stem cells will go for repair. Here is a demonstration of this procedure (see link at end of chapter).

6. The SPG is a site for intracranial penetration of the stem cells by stimulating insulin receptors on cell membranes. Now make a list such as Parkinson's, stroke, TBI, and the potential for treatment of other intracranial chronic diseases. Good judgment comes from experience.

7. Stem cells can be given intravenously for lung problems. Following the circulation from the intravenous administrative site in an arm, the blood first passes through the right side of the heart. The next path is through the lungs. The lung filters the blood at the alveolar capillary level. Then blood collects and goes back to the heart which pumps it out to the body. After leaving the heart many stem cells become sequestered in the spleen so their numbers diminish. But the first pass through the lungs makes this organ an easy target.

8. What can be added to an injection solution to help support the stem cells can be instrumental to promote a good results. This can include hyaluronic acid, low doses of bio identical hydrocortisone, growth hormone, and specific peptides to diminish inflammation and provide wound healing for the underlying condition treated.

9. Chronic inflammation influences stem cell activity by serving as a focus to attract stem cells. Chronic and severe inflammatory conditions produce a chemical called tumor necrosis factor (TNF). This is the real killer that causes damage with chronic inflammation. There are drugs that can block this effect. When this is given at the time of the stem cell injection it may influence the efficacy of the treatment. BPC 157 is commonly used for repair and regeneration.

10. As far as **systemic** administration of stem cells, there is no definite recipe that identifies specific <u>routine</u> measures that can be done to attract stem cells to areas of chronic inflammation for initiating their repair activity. Look at the notes above. This requires good judgment and experience on the part of the practitioner. The key is introducing an increase in blood supply which is the initial way the body localizes an area for healing.

11. During the procedure an MR4 low-level pulsed laser will be used. Focusing this light over various large blood vessels in the body can fully saturate the blood volume with nitric oxide. This helps stimulate stem cell activity.

12. Administration of stem cells has no significant risk and

can be administered conveniently.

13. This is not covered by insurance but I have seen many cases with favorable results better than those with conventional medicine. This is all about wound healing. Prepare the body and the body wants to heal itself.

One aspect of antiaging has to deal with parts that wear out. The patient can decide whether to promote as good healing as possible or have a joint replacement. Insurance policies cover joint surgery. To help you decide the best option, I try to put information out on the table in lay terms for patients to understand and to help them make a comfortable and personal decision.

Stem cells and the method with which they are administered can lead to impressive results, prevent surgery, and disable and repair some chronic processes.

******I reemphasize, **just injecting stem cells is not a complete procedure.**

https://www.youtube.com/watch?v=55lqZM_LVwg&feature=youtu.be

75

Personal Maintenance and Rejuvenation

- **Machines need repair and maintenance—how about us?**
- **NAD runs down just like everything else with aging.**
- **Exosomes can give you back youthful recovery.**
- **Epitalon can make you biologically younger.**
- **Telomeres are the yard marker to measure aging.**
- **Reboot your cells to function normally.**
- **Reversibility—the body wants to heal itself.**
- **Dr. Joe— pushing 70— body composition same as age 23.**

Machines need tuning and maintenance for optimum function. It is done for your car, boat, dishwasher, lawnmower, and other devices. How about personal maintenance?

Environmental exposure to plastics and toxins causes a premature drop in hormones leading to "accepted" aging.

This process can be slowed or reversed if the body is optimal for healing.

Areas such as nutrition are important for health. The source of nutrients is an even bigger key. On paper a patient may follow instructions such as eating salmon. If this is farm raised salmon it may be worthless or even harmful. Healthful nutrition can promote regeneration and healing but the organism needs to be ready to heal.

My experience with stem cells started 13 years ago when I found out that in age management body parts wear out. I started off injecting joints with retired NFL and NBA players.

I then got involved with military special operations workers. I used stem cells for injuries which included traumatic brain injury. The results led to treating MS patients with good results.

What I have seen in my 13 year experience with stem cell treatment is regeneration and healing. With a surgical background I use wound care principles including light and oxygen to promote healing which includes stem cell treatment. This is all about wound healing.

My observations and experience from the past 13 years has shown me that improving biologic function and administering stem cells can help things such as insulin resistance, blood pressure, energy levels, and libido. Patients treated systemically (such as emphysema and heart failure) rather than a joint injection have reported improvement in vision, use of reading glasses, and also hearing and taste. I have no specific explanation for this except that the overall biologic function of the human machine has improved. The body is healing itself.

Let us go to the next step—to reset the biologic clock. This can be important even if you think you are healthy. Get the cells to work normally. Our environment can be toxic. And body parts wear out.

The other thing to consider is the depletion of normal biochemicals in the cell that occur with age in a very subtle fashion with minimal symptoms. You do not need to go to the emergency room. For this reason this area is frequently ignored by conventional medicine and accepted by society that you are "just getting older." This can be reversed by restoring normal biologic chemicals rather than use something artificial.

See here a starting point I use for rebooting the body for each of my patients:

1. The first item is **NAD**— this represents nicotinamide adenine dinucleotide, which is a natural chemical particularly involved in the production of energy in the cell (the Krebs cycle which we all learned about in middle school biology). When energy production in the cell goes down the function of the cell degenerates. Thus the saying—" you are just getting older." Yet it can be reversible. NAD levels decrease with age and are significantly lower by age 50. Many chronic conditions lead to premature drop in NAD levels. With many chronic neurodegenerative conditions the nerve cells that are affected dump out all of their NAD. Then the nerve cells don't function properly and things such as neuropathies develop. These can be reversible. NAD is required in high levels for liver function (much depleted

with chronic alcohol use) and also for organs like the thyroid and pancreas. If NAD levels are down then the patient can develop a chronic degenerative condition. I have seen long-standing neurologic symptoms from various conditions improve immediately with intravenous NAD infusions. I follow with stem cell treatment because this improvement is not permanent. However, it demonstrates the importance of NAD levels and normal cell function.

2. **Exosomes** are natural biologic growth factors that improve the body's ability to heal itself. They stimulate stem cell activity. They can also be given alone without stem cells either by intravenous infusion or injected into a joint cavity. I have provided prolozone injections in the joints for many years. This has worked well but now it may be outdated many times. My experience with exosomes is that they are 100 times more effective than prolozone alone in joints. However, my program may consist of injection of exosomes and/or stem cells into a joint. Subsequently, less costly prolozone can be used at intervals to promote healing. I follow many of my patients with joint problems for two or three years minimum. I can still use it in that way. The cost of the exosomes and stem cells then is minimized.

3. Another step in approaching some joint as well as systemic diseases includes using **stem cells**. I will refer you to a gentleman by the name of Warren Osborn. At middle-age he developed symptoms compatible with ALS (amyotrophic lateral sclerosis). His initial treatment with stem cells also included hyperbaric oxygen treatments. I like this approach because the

thought process is right as far as wound healing. Mr. Osborn has improved and continues to follow an aggressive path since this is a highly deadly disease. Much of his progress also indicates that this is some sort of autoimmune condition.

4. I've seen a variety of significant systemic benefits after **exosomes alone** were given intravenously. This may include improvement in vision, less need for reading glasses, improvement in hearing, thickening and regrowth of hair, and one patient mentioned that taste had come back.

5. Another important aspect of rebooting cells is the use of **peptides**. These are small snips taken from a very large biologic protein giving a small protein called a peptide. Specific peptides have specific metabolic activities rather than the multiple functions seen with the large biologic protein. These can be given primarily for both general repair and regeneration.

6. **Epitalon** is a peptide (protein) that stimulates the pineal gland. The pineal in turn will physiologically tickle the hypothalamus and pituitary glands and so is involved with natural hormone production. It supports the immune system, has an anticancer property, and is a tremendous antioxidant. The pineal is involved with melatonin secretion which has to do with the day / night cycle or the circadian rhythm. This lifecycle is definitely involved with wound healing. As a surgeon I learned that wounds made earlier in the day had a better healing rate overall. Epitalon was patented by a Russian scientist 40 years ago. Most of the research with epitalon and aging is Russian resulting in

our conventional American medical system ignoring this. For me, however, the most significant factor is that epitalon is a very powerful agent to stimulate telomeres and to lengthen telomeres. If telomere length is increased then the patient becomes biologically younger.

Eight years ago my chronologic age was 62 and I had a biologic age of 56 measured using a telomere blood test. After this I followed a generally healthy program. I also did a personal maintenance rebooting and a 4 month course of epitalon. A year after epitalon with a chronologic age of 70 my biologic age was 54 using the same telomere measurement. Biologically younger (or same biologic age—that is okay too!).

A treatment course is about three days for the NAD infusion and exosomes. The epitalon is given as a subcutaneous injection for about 40 days and then it is discontinued. Consider repeating in six months or one year depending on any chronic or degenerative conditions present. Adding stem cells can take this to another level.

Finally, look at the prior chapter in this book on hydrogen water and dehydration. Another biologic step.

I have background and experience in both conventional as well as natural medicine. My observations with patients going through the above regimen include nails that grow twice as fast, hair becoming thicker with no gray, lowering of blood pressure, and increased energy. In many instances, after intravenous exosome injection patients relate that chronic low back pain present for many years definitely improved. Many soft tissue pains go away. Patients tell me they do not have to use reading glasses and that their hearing has become better. I also had a patient who told me he had not been able to taste food for 20 years. After the NAD treatment and exosomes he told me his taste was super.

I have seen insulin sensitivity improve. Prostate symptoms get better and libido goes way up.

This is just a matter of resetting and improving the ability of the body to heal. YOU ARE REBOOTING CELLS TO FUNCTION NORMALLY. The body wants to heal itself. Regeneration is rejuvenation. The process outlined is scientifically based. As a clinical scientist (physician) I have learned to listen to my patients. Experience promotes better judgment.

In my experience I have seen improvement in many patients using the above treatment plan.

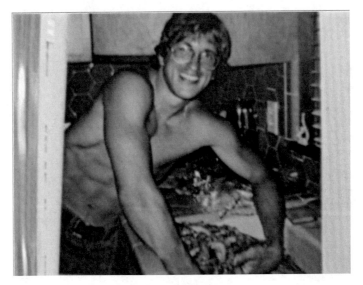

Doc Joe at age 23

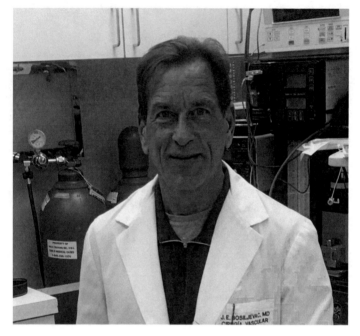

Doc Joe at 70 years old

So this is my contention:

1. At the age of 50, even if you feel healthy, develop good baseline data that can help direct a program and also indicate how aggressive this should be.
2. Next, take a patient with multiple symptoms secondary to an autoimmune condition. They may have 10 different specialists and multiple treatments such as physical therapy. This patient undergoes a rejuvenation program resulting in cells that work more normal. Many symptoms will disappear. The patient is re-

assessed and at that point a more specific and simplified program can be presented to the patient since many of the specialists are not needed.

3. 150 years ago a doctor would go to the patient's home and stay with the patient during the illness. The doctor is taking personal control and decision-making even into the patient's home. This is Back to the Future medicine. I have been seeing patients on their own turf, comfortable and convenient.

Some final reference sites are listed below. Please follow us on the our continuing journey towards health and longevity.

www.DrJBoss.com

Facebook: New York Health and Longevity

https://www.youtube.com/watch?v=4FmP1zzyDsA&feature=youtu.be 5 minute video

https://vimeo.com/289141444

www.cenegenics-drbosiljevac.com

http://www.empowereddoctor.com/dr-joe-bosiljevac-anti-aging-and-integrative-medicine

https://www.blogtalkradio.com/physicianinc/2019/09/19/autoimr and-exosomes-with-join-joseph-e-bosiljevac-jr-md-phd-facs

https://player.fm/series/herbally-yours/how-to-approach-longevity

https://www.youtube.com/watch?v=fU35gpn3Ubw

http://r3stemcell.com/nyc/ny/anti-aging/

https://vimeo.com/114403798 Password: ginseng

76

Back to the Future by Corbin Bosiljevac

Recently I had the privilege of accompanying my father on some meetings and therapies with patients. I have been doing this on and off over the course of my life, growing up with someone being as busy as he was with his medical businesses. I did not follow him in to the medical field, but have always had involvement in the health and medicinal aspect of life.

Interestingly, I was able to assist in 2 different stem cell procedures. Up close, I was able to see the process of administering the meds and natural therapies while getting the satisfaction of helping improve the lives of individuals. But most significantly was when we met with these people about their situations. We discussed with them their quality of life and their yearning for something better for themselves. Better health for them meant a better life.

You see, I have always known my father to keep the best interests of his patients at the forefront of the services he provides. Mind, body, and spirit must all be in the most comfortable place in order to get the maximum effects of healing. As we have seen, 2020 has brought numerous difficulties for humans to overcome. Just because a pandemic hit and many businesses were forced to close for a chunk of time didn't meant that the health of people was to be put on hold. Quite the opposite I would say! Now, health was more important that ever.

Several years ago in Manhattan my father began the practice of making house calls. High profile patients with busy schedules appreciated that he would see them at their house, workplace, hotel, or wherever was most convenient for them. He made it a point to work around their schedules in order to keep health as a key aspect in these people's lives. It was important to them and so it was important to my father.

With travel being difficult in 2020, New York became a place that people were leaving instead of flocking to. With that in mind, he decided to embrace the idea of making house calls and take his practice on the road. He had a few patients needing stem cell procedures in Ohio so he obtained a license there and traveled to his patients instead of suggesting to them the inconvenience of traveling during a pandemic.

This is where his theory of "Back to the Future" comes in. By going back to the way that doctor's used to practice in making house calls and carrying around the black doctor's bag, he was pivoting his practice to fit the times.

Why not go to the patient? Especially if the patient is quite ill or isn't comfortable traveling to New York City, the epicenter of the coronavirus in 2020. By continuing to be forward thinking with his practice and passing on his wealth of knowledge, he is using old methods from 100 years ago to modernize his clinic. For the patient to be ready to heal they must be in the most comfortable state of being, considering mind, body and spirit.

This is the philosophy of New York Health and Longevity, the practice that Doc Joe runs today in Manhattan, New York. To see what is best for the patient and the situation at hand and do whatever is possible to get the desired results. I always thought that if more medical professionals had this approach to their patients then humanity would be better off and more healthy. Then also, that is what has afforded my father an unique and successful career.

Enjoy the final two chapters of this book. They offer the beginnings of advice from some very knowledgeable people that are good at what they do. The quest for good health is a journey and the starting point is different for every person. Just make sure you are moving forward in your quest and on to the next thing!

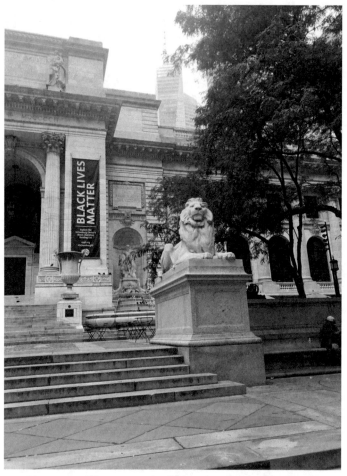

Lions, the library, and a hint of social justice in the foreshadow of the Freedom Tower. Under one lion is labeled patience, under the other fortitude. Which one do you see here?

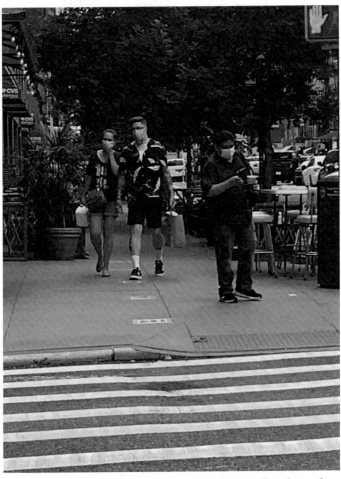

Outdoor seating has helped restaurants survive these slow months in the middle of 2020.

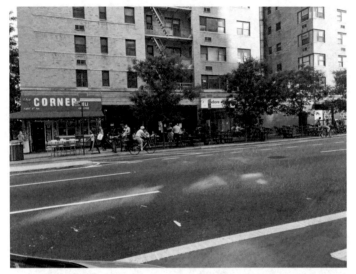

Cold weather and continued shutdowns threaten the service industry going into the fall of 2020.

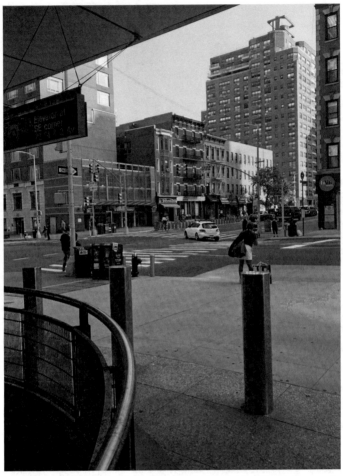

Street and pedestrian traffic is less than half of it's usual hustle and bustle.

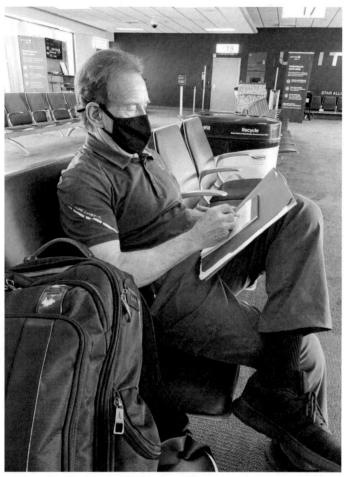

Doc Joe traveling to Ohio, working his 'back to the future'
approach.

77

Exercise at Home: A Personal Program

During the Corona pandemic no gyms have been open. Many of my patients stated that they took a break from exercising and their health program during the pandemic.

I have maintained the same weight the past few years with about 10% total body fat. This is the same body composition when I was 23. People comment that I must work out a lot. My workout consists of about 15 minutes four times a week. My cardio is climbing 12 flights of stairs without stopping while carrying a 30 pound weight jacket. I do this to achieve my peak heart rate of 160. That partakes five minutes. Add 10 minutes body weight resistance exercise and I'm done. Resistance is important to maintain and increase muscle mass.

There is no excuse for not exercising. I have executives that travel and say they don't have time for the gym because are so busy at work. 50 push-ups, 50 sit ups, and a few other body weight exercises and climbing stairs can easily be added to a very busy working routine. Just a few minutes.

It is important to monitor body composition. People lose weight but there may be more muscle mass loss than fat. This is not healthy.

This chapter is from my brother who is a retired US Navy SEAL and working as a special operations member now. He may be deployed for three months where his lifestyle and discipline changes on deployment take a toll as far as eating and exercise. By maintaining a personal workout routine, he is able to keep up a fairly healthy lifestyle.

In addition, there is a note from a chief medical officer, Dr. Rand McClain, who works with my brother. He reports on healthy aspects of an East African tribe called the Hazda.

Time spent in moderate-to-vigorous physical activity (MVPA) is a strong predictor of cardiovascular health, yet few humans living in industrialized societies meet current recommendations (150 min/week). Researchers have long suggested that human physiological requirements for aerobic exercise reflect an evolutionary shift to a hunting and gathering foraging strategy, and a recent transition to more sedentary lifestyles likely represents a mismatch with our past in terms of physical activity. The goal of this study is to explore this mismatch by characterizing MVPA and cardiovascular health in the Hadza, a modern hunting and gathering population living in Northern Tanzania.

https://onlinelibrary.wiley.com/doi/10.1002/ajhb.22919

This has to do with keeping your muscles active even when you are resting. The key here is just get out of the chair and do a little walking intermittently during the day.

He reports that this tribe would spend most of their days

resting and are very healthy. The secret is they keep their muscles active even when the resting. They do a full squat or rest on their knees when they sit down.

As far as the United States, the one simple fix can give you the same benefits. Stand up every 30 minutes and walk a little bit. This even gives a little advantage to a standing desk.

Overtraining can affect the immune system. Consider the article below.

https://www.runnersworld.com/health-injuries/a32268595/how-running-affects-your-immune-system/

It has been shown that social distancing when running should be more like 30 feet because of the transmission of virus with heavy breathing.

https://www.runnersworld.com/health-injuries/a32268595/how-running-affects-your-immune-system/

Using caution while exercising during a pandemic is important. Here is a nice summary of how to run safely amid coronavirus concerns.

https://www.runnersworld.com/news/a31439358/running-during-coronavirus/

My current exercise routine is for the maintenance of regular life. If I plan another wilderness camping trip that can be more physically demanding then I would train more seriously for 4 to 6 weeks prior to the trip.

This was sent to me by my brother. Remember, he is a retired US Navy SEAL and is quite disciplined and dedicated to his craft. We thank him for his service and continued dedication to our country —

Joe, here's some exercises & fitness concepts that I utilize:

Always go the power route, but use bodyweight.

https://www.studyfinds.org/lifting-weights-can-lead-longer-life-not-weight-exercises-equal/

As an example, ever try Superman pushups? They're awesome and will make you powerful and quick. Check the last third of this video.

https://www.youtube.com/watch?v=9YKiXIuFHF0

It's all in the imagination - all bodyweight

https://www.youtube.com/watch?v=ilh-78AaSjQ

1. FITNESS is defined by the individual. Many variables depending on age, capabilities, goals, etc...

I have a lot of things I work on for my personal fitness. That frames my choice of exercises, number of sets, repetitions, order of exercise construction, etc... So when I outline or describe some of the exercises below, I do them for me and my goals. They may or may not work for others, but there will be value in studying them and why I do them. I'm not into balance balls and all kinds of exotic gear. I'll only hurt myself on that stuff.

Some of my goals include strength, aerobic & anaerobic fitness, lactic acid threshold increase, flexibility, fighting skill without weapons, fighting skill with weapons, mobility, agility, coordination, speed, tempo, and overall health. I train like a mixed martial artist. Want to be strong, but not big muscles that burn a lot of oxygen. Lots of interval training. Lots of sprints. Hard, short resistance training to boost T levels & HGH naturally. I also want to do things that I never outgrow – I want to be able to do more and get stronger or in better condition. Also, for resistance work, intensity is key. The less time you do something, the more intensity you use for better results.

2. I work hard not to incur an injury.

Injuries screw your schedule up and hold you back. Additionally, injuries are trauma to your body, and your body has to process that trauma. That's lost time and energy. I do a lot of things that make me move, but I stay mostly linear in my movements, cutting down on the odds of getting a tear or joint injury. I do a few exercises to prepare my body for impacts, such as what takes place when you fall down. (I do a Judo type roll as part of my warm up – learned it while taking Aikido, and I feel it helps tremendously). So instead of playing tennis (lots of cutting around) or playing pick up basketball or football, I do my own fitness stuff.

3. That said, I work on a lot of bodyweight stuff.

I have to be CONSISTENT in my workouts, and traveling a lot does not always allow me to have equipment. I have to have exercises to do in transit. Also, you have to be able to measure for improvements and to be able to adjust workouts. Doing some of the same exercises and recording results will give you that measure. The more meticulous you measure, the better info you will have to motivate you, just as being meticulous in your diet will provide health improvements.

Here's some exercises:

Body Weight Bench Press – Regular bench press without overloading the bar for an injury. If you can do 15 good reps in a single set, you're looking good on "push" strength….the type of strength used to strike someone. I recently did a personal best ever of 22 without doing any type of weight lifting routine to work up for it.

Hindu Push Up – Learned from Matt Furey, a former Mixed Martial Artist.

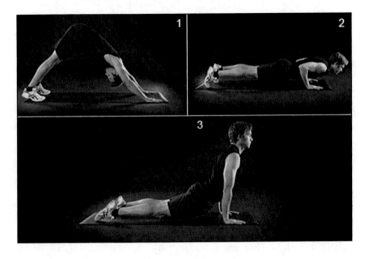

Place your feet (shoulder width or wider) and palms on the floor in a downward-facing-dog yoga pose. In one fluid movement, drop down into push-up position, roll up into an upward-facing-dog pose, then reverse and return to start.

I like to go with a very wide foot stance, as wide as I can get them. Just dip down face first, then chest, etc.....until you arch with your arms locked and legs almost on the floor. Reverse it to get to starting position. This thing rocks. It will shred your shoulders, pecs, and triceps big time, and your cardio will be wasted. Great for the spine. Work until you can get a single set of 100 without stopping. Then start working a set of 100 in 4 minutes or less. I do these a lot. My best time ever was 2:35...I maintain about a 2:50-55 average currently. Great striking and muscular endurance exercise.

Inverted Press – Do a handstand balancing against a wall. Start at arms length. Bend arms until the top of your head contacts the ground, then push back to arms length.5 is looking good. 5+ is real good. Again, striking strength.

Chin Ups – Find a bar or other device, get a close grip over your head, palms facing you. Let yourself hang, pull until your chin goes over the bar, then return to a hang. This is the "Squat" of the upper body. Arthur Jones who invented the Nautilus machine years ago felt this was the most perfect exercise for the biceps. This strengthens the "Pulling" muscles of the body used for grappling and choking people out. Great for grip, biceps, lats. 15 is good. I did a single set of 31 this week as part of a workout. I'm starting to wonder if I could actually get to 50........

AB "V" – Sit on the floor. Keeping your legs straight, point your toes & raise your legs off the ground until they are at a 45 degree angle off the ground. Lean your upper body back, but keep it off the ground, extending your arms straight ahead and parallel to the ground for balance. Your only contact with the ground will be in the area of your tailbone. Hold that of 60 seconds. Great ab and core exercise.

Pistols – Essentially a full squat and return while balanced on one leg. Great for balance and strength. Not recommended for those with damaged knees. Fantastic exercise. Some guys are strong enough to do them while holding a kettlebell or dumbbell in front of their chest. When you can get to more than 5 consecutively in a single set, you're doing awesome.

468

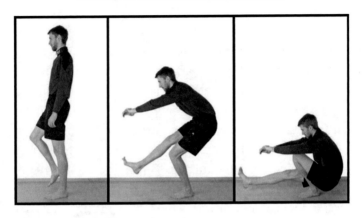

Plyometric Jumps – A box jump without the box. I can't take a box with me, and I don't want to chance missing a jump and jamming a shin into the side of a box or falling over (I've seen some guys sustain some serious damage doing that.) I found a few things. First, I went to a professional course for some rehab that was manned by people who work with Olympic and professional athletes. They taught me that for warm ups, you need to increase blood flow and muscle warmth, but also warm up and awaken the neuro system. I found they were right. They used a moderately heavy dumbbell for snatches (from the side to overhead in a single fluid but explosive move.) I also found from an article I read and tried, that doing some extra plyometric jumps in my workout increased work volume for my legs, the biggest muscles in the body that can handle more load. So here's what I started doing, and it works like a champ.

As part of warm-ups, I intersperse 5 plyometric jumps with some hip loosening work and breathing exercises. I do the same during my cooldown. I do it differently for those two times to help my coordination. During warmup jumps, I start hands by my side. I squat down as far as I can go, look down, and extend my arms forward and up. Without hesitation at the bottom of the squat, I explode and jump up as physically hard and far as I can, bringing my arms down hard. When I land, I bend at the knees to soften my landing.

During my cooldowns, I do it differently. I start arms extended overhead, looking up, I squat down to full depth while bringing my arms down and to the rear. Without hesitation, I explode upward while throwing my arms first up high, then down to my sides as I reach full extension. Each jump is done all out, as if trying a record. Momentary all out intensity is required.

I do one other plyo jump during the course of stretching at the end of a workout, just for agility. I bounce off the ground a few times, then jump up as high off the ground as I can and touch my knees to my chest, wrapping my arms around my shins momentarily.

All the plyo jumps are easy and as you get stronger and in better shape, you'll feel powerful and agile.

Neck Bridge – This has really helped my back and spine, but I don't do it for a long period of time. Get on your back, bridge up on your head and feet, shift immediately to up on the very tips of your toes (not flat footed) and arch. Try to imagine touching your forehead to the ground….that's how hard you should arch. The biggest strain should be rock hard glutes, pushing your pelvis skyward. Hold that for as long as you wish. I do a 30 second bridge as part of a series of all my skills work every day.

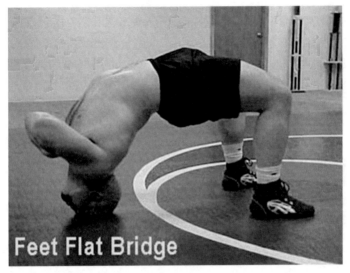

Feet Flat Bridge

That's Matt Furey in the photo, although I couldn't find a good one of him up on his toes.

Ring Dips & Rig Chins – Just like a gymnast, but you have to buy a set or have them at the gym. I was shocked at how difficult they were at first, but they truly increase strength tremendously. I do them every week now. Dips executed just like on parallel bars, chins just like on a bar. When you can do more than 10 full dips, you're getting there. My best is 22 so far. Chins the same. I can do more than 15 now. Great for push & pull strength and power.

Dips – Just mount a set of parallel bars and hit it. Full dip is when the upper arms are bent 90 degrees or better. SEALs easily knock out sets of 30 in training.

Kettlebell Training – Old school Russian exercise. The "HINGE" motion is key to all athleticism and sports. Bend at the knees & squat down slightly, bend forward at the waist, push ass back a little, then snap your body upright. Coaches & trainers measure potential by vertical jumps, which measure this hinge motion. It's in all the combines.

The kettlebell works that hinge motion like a Shetland pony at a little kid's birthday party. Kettlebells come in all different weights, and their popularity has made them available in most sports stores. Lots of exercises for coordination, explosive power, strength, stamina. Very functional. Here's some

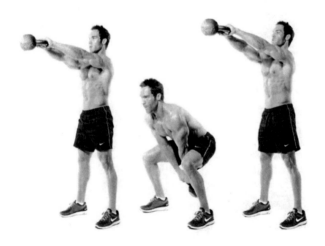

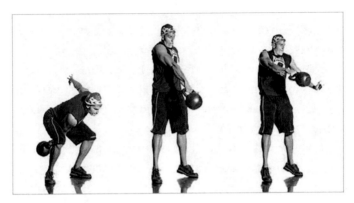

Two and One Handed Swing

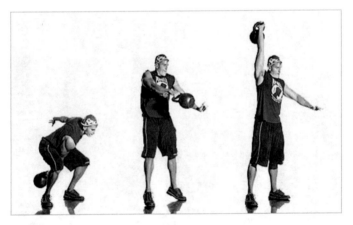

Snatch

There are all kinds of exercises and routines that absolutely rip you and increase work and cardio capacities like a furnace. There are guys that are so good at this stuff, they actually flip the kettlebells in the air as they do the workout to increase their power, hand and eye coordination, and agility. Can't out live this one....just get the next biggest kettlebell. Go online and check it out. Almost everyone who does these for any length of time is ripped!

Enough for now. Hope this is of some help. For some of you this may appear excessive. What I am trying to present are a few simple examples of methods to maintain muscle strength and flexibility.

It is always an individual program. Like a health coach I try to give good advice. You take it from there.

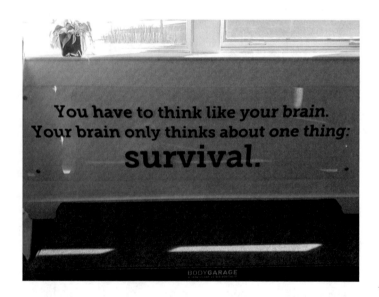

78

Diet

Diet is considered a big part of health, I would say 80% or more. This is an article published in the American Journal of clinical nutrition.

A study demonstrated that patients who consume a lot of industrial processed junk foods are more likely to exhibit a change in chromosomes linked to aging. This has to do with the telomeres and telomere length.

Industrial foods that are nutritionally poor are composed of a mix of oils, fats, sugars, starch, and proteins that contain very little if any whole or natural foods. They will also include artificial flavorings, emulsifiers, preservatives, coloring, and other additives to increase shelf life.

I have been using a doctor out of the University of Navarra Spain to do telomere testing on my patients for many years. Their measurement will give you a biologic age to compare with your chronological age.

In this study nearly 900 patients who were 55 years of age or older provided DNA samples in 2008 and provided detailed data about eating habits at that time as well as every two years afterwards. Participants taking large amounts of processed foods had <u>definite increased shortening</u> of the telomeres when they were measured 10 years later. They were getting old faster!

Preservation of telomeres and prevention of DNA degradation that may occur with some things such as smoking, x-ray exposure, and other environmental factors has been accepted. In addition, there is a strong correlation between ultra-processed food and obesity, type II diabetes, hypertension, depression, and some types of cancer. This has <u>not</u> been presented publicly.

Take a shoestring and hold it out in front with both hands. This represents a DNA strand. The little plastic 'aglets' on both ends that protect stability of the DNA (shoestring) during reproduction represent telomeres. Each time the DNA strand replicates, these aglets prevent unraveling of the ends of the DNA strand.

I have promoted the personal maintenance program that actually restores or reboots cells back to more optimal function.

Telomeres are good measurements to reflect biologic age. In this regard telomeres may be preserved or sometimes with the use of a peptide called <u>epitalon</u> may actually increase in length. That makes a patient biologically younger!

I have one patient who eight years ago had a baseline chronological age of 62 and a biologic age of 56 using telomere measurement. A health program for 8 years was followed including a year of epitalon. In follow up at a chronologic age of 70, the patient's biologic age was 54 using the same telomere measurement. Biologically the same or younger. This is me.

I am not going to give you a chapter on nutrition. There are better experts out there than me. But, I will give you a few key things to look at.

First of all follow a whole food concept. When patients go to the grocery store I tell them to come out without any boxes, packages, cans, or bottles. Several patients have commented if they did that they would not have any groceries.

The next aspect is the food source. Fruits and vegetables may be picked before ripe. Depending on the environment and where they were raised they may lack certain trace minerals. And how organic is organic? Always a question. Just do the best you can.

As far as animal products you want wild. Red beef that is grass fed is very healthy versus the feedlot corn fed cattle. Farm raised salmon is not the same as wild.

And just stay away from processed food. Even if on paper the food appears nutritious, the source and the way it is prepared can be unhealthy. Most restaurants use canola oil, which was originally patented in Canada in the 1940s as a pesticide. Enough said.

A final comment would be that of processed water. Natural water has a reasonably high hydrogen concentration. This is the hydrogen from a water molecule that becomes dissolved in solution and has a lot to do as far as intracellular hydration and the assimilation of trace minerals into the cell. The two parts of hydration are water and trace minerals. "Water–It May Be Almost Everywhere But Not Good Everywhere" **and** "Dehydration".

First start with **water**. Glass is a very viscous or thick liquid and is formed by a crystalline structure. This allows transparency through the glass. Water should also form a good liquid crystalline structure. What do I mean by this?

This can be measured in different ways. Sometimes the angle of the molecular connection between the oxygen and hydrogen in the water molecule can affect how water molecules interact with each other. If the phase angle is appropriate this allows the water molecules to align into a nice crystalline structure. "Hydrating at the Cellular Level," this structure enables passage of the water and minerals into the cell. Acid-base levels or pH, electrical conduction, and even magnetic fields can potentially affect the crystalline structure of the water. 5G may be a potential problem—a recent study shows it causes viruses to mutate. It may also affect water structure.

This is not simply a matter of buying spring water or purified water. Source, preparation, transportation, and contaminants may be involved with aspects that could affect the health benefit of water. Certainly, municipal processed water is completely disorganized. As such, it has a decreased ability to penetrate cells and transport substances back and forth.

Think about the whole food concept as far as diet. Nutrient content can be deficient after processing whole food into a box or a can. Processed food is not healthy. What I refer to above is **processed water** when structure is changed. It is a process that can occur in healthy water stored in plastic bottles, for example.

1. Currently there has been an increasing interest in hydrogen water with respect to increasing proper hydration inside the cell. Water, which is a combination

of one oxygen and two hydrogen atoms, has a dissolved portion of hydrogen gas in the water in the concentration of about 0.6 ppm (parts per million). This is the normal status of unprocessed water. Nobody has touched it yet. After processing, it degrades further. Many times, the amount of dissolved hydrogen in processed water we drink is in the range of 0.08 ppm.

2. Most water we all drink to "keep hydrated" is WORTHLESS—well, let me say significantly suboptimal. Natural water has a normal crystalline structure that enables many of the electromagnetic properties of our body. This structure degrades with processing of water. It also degrades with environmental electromagnetic influences such as cell phones. Very subtle but this can affect our biologic function. The majority of water we drink is suboptimal to promote healing— actually, it barely sustains us. It slowly degrades and requires considerable energy to restore the normal crystalline structure of water. That's right, the concept of you're getting older' is accepted. Hydrogen helps us rebuild the crystalline structure of water—that is on the bottom line to restore longevity.

3. Therapeutic effects of hydrogen water has been demonstrated by the Japanese since 2007. It is absorbed through the intestines within one minute and spreads through the entire body in ten. Hydroxyl (-OH) and lipid radicals are erased.

4. There are magnesium tablets that can be dropped into a bottle of water that increase the part per million (ppm) concentration of hydrogen dissolved in water. Some companies claim their product can increase the

concentration to 10 ppm. Bottled prepared hydrogen water is not as potent, maybe more the range of 1-2 ppm.

5. If you look at my own K/Na ratio I show mild intracellular dehydration with the ratio of 0.31. I have eight years data. This never increased even though I was ingesting more water. I began drinking 3 or 4 of 8 ounce glasses of hydrogen water daily. I prepared this with tablets that make a concentration of 10 ppm dissolved hydrogen in the water. The dissolved hydrogen will make the water opaque. If it is drank immediately it is absorbed from the intestine within one minute and diffuses throughout the body over 10 minutes. If left alone the opaque water will become clear again as the hydrogen evaporates. Over 2 years my K/Na ratio improved to 0.45.

6. Is it valid? Yes, and I speak from the aspect of improving the natural ability of the body to function better and heal itself using water that has increased dissolved hydrogen. Look at the detoxification of oxidized radicals. The -OH group encounters a hydrogen atom (H) and forms water (H_2O). Hydrogen serves to detoxify oxidized lipid radicals as well as chemicals and preservatives like hydrogen sulfide in processed food. Reboot. Personal maintenance.

1 October 2020

- As I finish this, President Trump just entered Walter Reed Hospital with some minor symptoms of Corona. The non-health consequences have hit this country hard during this current election.

- My doorman can park in the building garage for free. Management wants them to stay away from the subway.
- One of my patients recently spent a weekend in a hotel in Newport, Rhode Island. The hotel was limited for social distancing but still open, and restaurants there have been open on a limited basis.
- Restaurant business is down here in NYC.
- Many businesses are slow. Everyone has learned to order online.
- I see a few patients but there still are others that are very reluctant to come out of hiding. Everyone is so fearful of the current pandemic.
- Nursing homes restrict visitors. In community centers for older people activities such as bingo are on hold.
- I was planning to use this as a stop point for this book. I am anxious to see if the predicted incidence of the Asian flu virus and a second peak of COVID-19 occurs. Hopefully, that will show we have gained some as a society to confront a pandemic. There could be more to come.
- This may have been planned.
- Trump received a sympathy call from President of China.
- Be safe.

https://worldhealth.net/news/study-links-junk-food-age-marker-chromosomes/

79

Final Thoughts

10 October 2020

We are dealing with a virus, and viruses will never be totally eliminated from our environment. Temporary measures are just a bridge to give our society time to assess the situation and realize a more permanent strategy. We have never accumulated this amount of testing data regarding incidence and spread with any virus before.

The truth is this: viruses will propagate until sufficient population has active antibodies against it. Sooner or later it continues to spread. With time and the accumulation of antibodies in most people, the virus spread and incidence will decrease. This can occur with continued spread or also with antibodies from a vaccination. This is called "herd immunity."

The "second wave" of COVID-19 may demonstrate increased incidence but less morbidity if we protect nursing homes, handicapped, and the elderly. Much of the mortality with the current wave of coronavirus may have been because we were not prepared as individuals or as a society for something like this. When people compare this to 9/11, corona ravages can be severe but perhaps this pandemic is worse because of our response.

Current methods are killing business, social relations, family relationships, and our overall way of life. The temporary measures we put into place are becoming more normalized. It is time to think beyond these temporary measures and consider the many more permanent measures as discussed in this book. All of which deal with making personal health a priority.

Fear is being propagated by the media. Restrictions bear down on businesses and schools in certain districts because the incidence is "too high."

This is all part of a big soap opera in our country. We try to slow down the propagation of the virus yet it continues slowly despite all the businesses and relationships that have deteriorated to nothing. By delaying the spread, the distress on society is also prolonged.

It is important to give ourselves a chance. A chance again at freedom and at choice. These two things are what has made our society great for generations. If we can choose to be healthier today than we were yesterday, then we are certainly giving ourselves that chance.

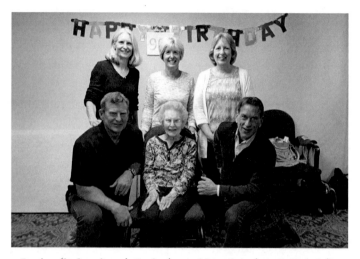

Janice (baby sister), Judy (my older sister) and Carol (in between but younger), Tim (3 years younger), mom age 90 (now deceased), me. Photo taken in 2017.

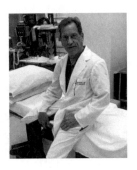

About the Author

Dr. Joseph Bosiljevac is a descendant from Croatian immigrants and has spent his entire career learning how to optimize the use of the human machine. Always on the cutting edge of medicine, he consistently keeps safety and the well-being of each patient at his highest regard. He loves seeing people's quality of life improve and has the lofty goal of living actively past age 100 himself.

Besides his print and radio media involvement, his accolades include earning his MD and PhD as well as being a member of the Fellow American College of Surgeons. He currently resides on the Upper East Side of Manhattan, NY and has offices on 79th St. and in the Trump Building on Wall Street.

Doc Joe has 4 children. His son, Corbin, assists him in his writings and various other management aspects of his business endeavors. Corbin puts personal health at the center of everything he does and sees combating the world as a mission that each individual must endure. His other children are Tyler, Dr. Kristin and Laura

You can connect with me on:

🌐 https://www.drjboss.com

📘　https://www.facebook.com/New-York-Health-and-Longevity-106487457845708/notifications

✒ https://www.facebook.com/Blu-Press-Media-104015661482469